NEUROSCIENCE RESEARCH PROGRESS

HANDEDNESS: THEORIES, GENETICS AND PSYCHOLOGY

NEUROSCIENCE RESEARCH PROGRESS

Additional books in this series can be found on Nova's website under the Series tab.

Additional E-books in this series can be found on Nova's website under the E-books tab.

NEUROSCIENCE RESEARCH PROGRESS

HANDEDNESS: THEORIES, GENETICS AND PSYCHOLOGY

JAMES DUNHAM
AND
TODD DAVENPORT
EDITORS

Nova Science Publishers, Inc.
New York

For permission to use material from this book please contact us:
Telephone 631-231-7269; Fax 631-231-8175
Web Site: http://www.novapublishers.com

Library of Congress Cataloging-in-Publication Data

Handedness : theories, genetics, and psychology / editors, James Dunham and Todd Davenport.
p. cm.
Includes bibliographical references and index.
ISBN 978-1-61470-502-4 (hardcover : alk. paper) 1. Left- and right-handedness. I. Dunham, James, 1962- II. Davenport, Todd.
QP385.5.H36 2011
152.3'35--dc23

2011023190

Published by Nova Science Publishers, Inc. † New York

Contents

Preface

Handedness is an attribute of humans defined by their unequal distribution of fine motor skill between the left and right hands. A minority of people are equally skilled with both hands, and are termed ambidextrous. This book presents current research in the study of handedness, including the significance of knot-tying habits in handedness research and forensic science; manual laterality and hemispheric specialization for language; handedness and mental rotation; handedness and achievement in sports and handedness of children determines preferential facial and eye movements.

Chapter I – Questionnaires, skill assessments – such as the Edinburgh and Briggs-Nebes Handedness Inventories – association analysis, brain scans, and other methods have been instrumental in a variety of research interests. A range of uni-manual preferences have been identified. Handedness, popularly assessed according to writing preferences, is not binary or one-dimensional. Evolving from Piaget's early work and epistemology, as well as traditional and experiential knotting acumen, the analysis of innate knot-tying habits is an esoteric field concerned with class-characteristic evidence in forensic science. Most relevant, focussed empirical investigations have yielded an analogous spectrum of preferences in one-wend and two-wend tying tasks – from the dominance of the more prevalent S enantiomers, which are strongly associated with dextrality, to the opposite or Z chiral form. Data and theoretical models linking handedness and tying habits are discussed, along with speculations regarding the potential in profiling tying habits and the importance of noting knot chirality in future research.

Chapter II – Manual asymmetry has long fascinated investigators, and the rarity of left-handed individuals in the general population has been a puzzle. Researchers have endeavoured to answer three fundamental questions: What is handedness? How can it be measured? What are its mechanisms? These questions delve into the very nature of brain function and they have served to guide psychologists, educators, physicians, therapists, physiologists and other scientists in their quest to unravel numerous mysteries. What follows is a brief historical outline of theories that gave rise to current behavioural, genetic, and physiological models of laterality and handedness.

Chapter III – The aim of this article is to describe ancient and modern theories of human laterality based on recent data on manual and cerebral specialization. Manual specialization and handedness are distinct manifestations of manual laterality. Handedness results from genetic, environmental, pathological, and activity-related factors, and their interactions. Manual specialization is a more direct manifestation of cerebral specialization than handedness. In young infants and in nonhuman primates, most of researches have demonstrated a manual specialization. Questions concerning measurement, uni- or multidimensionality, plasticity and activity-related factors, sex differences, or age effect, are common for the two domains, manual laterality and cerebral specialization, illustrating the strong link between manual gestures and language.

Chapter IV – Right-handed and left-handed individuals have been found to differ in their ability to perform tasks with the dominant and non-dominant hand. Laterality of brain function in verbal tasks and spatial cognitive tasks also appears to differ according to handedness. Spatial cognitive tasks involving mental rotation of shapes have been used to study the relationships of handedness, handedness of immediate family and sex to reaction time and correct response rate. Cerebral activation during these tasks has also been studied. The relationship between handedness and reaction time has also been investigated in tasks involving mental rotation of hand images, where the subject is presented with a photograph or drawing of a hand rotated at a specific angle and must judge whether it is a left or right hand. Authors have previously published studies on brain activation during the mental rotation of shapes and on reaction times in the mental rotation of hand pictures in left- and right-handed subjects. In this paper authors review the literature relating to the relationship of handedness to reaction times and brain activation in mental rotation tasks.

Chapter V – A finger tapping task was employed to investigate fine motor performance rate by healthy adult right (RH) and left (LH) handers in right versus left hemispace. Eighty healthy adults tapped rapidly with the right or left hand index finger during uncued, unpaced, uni- and bimanual conditions. Two strikingly significant results emerged: (1.) The right hand showed a significant effect of space, but the left hand did not; this irrespective of handedness or number of hands employed. (2.) This effect of space favoured the right side. Overall, these findings support fMRI and lesion evidence indicating that side of space influences the extent of motor asymmetry. The result is novel and shows an effect which is independent of hand preference; that is, right versus left handedness.

Chapter VI – Marc Dax is thought to have been the first to propose the doctrine of cerebral dominance, a model in which the faculty of language is controlled by the cerebral hemisphere contralateral to the preferred hand. Then, Broca and Wernicke described left hemispheric language dominance based on their anatomo- pathological findings in patients who presented clinically with aphasic disturbances. Since the 19th century, handedness has been associated with language dominance, though "Broca's rule" has been challenged by clinical and functional imaging studies, no latter than soon after its emergence and the brain representation of language in the right hemisphere still remains controversial. To evaluate the role of handedness in language lateralization, authors investigated 50 patients harboring right-sided brain tumors. There were 17 left-handers (33%) 33 right-handers (66%), who ranged in age from 22 to 78 years (mean: 50.4 years). These patients were all operated on using awake craniotomy procedures (i.e., their language was intraoperatively mapped by electrostimulation mapping prior to tumor resection). Overall, 814 of 824 cortical sites (98.8%) were not associated with stimulation induced language deficit (Pre- and post-central gyri sensori-motor sites inferring with articulatory process of language were excluded from the analysis). Nevertheless, 8 of the 50 patients (16%) had at least one site where stimulation disrupted language function. Authors found that 4 out of 17 left-handers (23.5%) had positive language maps in their dominant hemisphere, whereas 4 out of 33 right-handers (12.2%) had positive language maps in their non-dominant hemisphere. This stimulation mapping series is the largest ever-published one on the right hemisphere language mapping. Electrostimulation can detect non-motor language sites in the right hemisphere of left- but also right-handed patients although this is rare. Further exploratory studies are needed in the future to evaluate the clinical significance of RH naming sites and the possible aetiologies of the "atypical" localization of these language sites. Once, awake surgery could be useful to detect and spare language areas in some patients when surgery is considered in right hemisphere.

Chapter VII – Handedness is a preference for the use of one of the right- or the left-hands. In the large majority of right-handers, speech is controlled by the left side of the brain. Also, the right hemisphere of the brain is usually specialized for recognizing and remembering faces and understanding relationships in space. Authors live in a right-handed world and that left-handers have an inherent disadvantage in using tools designed for right-handers. Left-handed persons are believed to have better developed motor, attentional and spatial functions. Some studies have explored a possible correlation between left-handedness and enhanced performance in specific sports such as baseball, cricket, fencing, soccer and tennis. The rate of the left-handed boxers was higher compared to the right-handed ones in the National Road Sport Men Boxing Club in Turkey. These results may be associated with two suggestions: 1. the left-handed subjects have an intrinsic advantage over right-handers due to superior spatio-motor skills, 2. advantage in the left-handed boxer and the left-handed other athletes may result from the nature of the game (boxing) or frequency-dependent strategic advantage.

Chapter VIII – Despite repeated demonstrations of asymmetries in several brain functions, the biological bases of such asymmetries have remained obscure The objective of study was to investigate development of lateralized facial and eye movements evoked by hemispheric stimulation in right-handed and left-handed children. Fifty children were tested according to handedness by four tests: I. Mono-syllabic non-sense words, II. Tri-syllabic sense words, III. Visual field occlusion by black wall, and presentation of geometric objects to both hands separatelly, IV. Left eye and the temporal half visual field of the right eye occlusion with special goggles, afterwards asking children to assemble a three-piece puzzle; same tasks were performed contralaterally. Right-handed children showed higher percentage of eye movements to right side when stimulated by tri-syllabic words, while left-handed children shown higher percentages of eyes movements to left side when stimulated by tri-syllabic words. Left-handed children spent more time in recognizing mono-syllabic words. Hand lateralitycorrelated with tri-syllabic word recognition performance. Age contributed to laterality development in nearly all cases, except in second test. *Conclusions:* Eye and facial movements were found to be related to left- and right-hand preference and specialization for language development, as well as visual, haptic perception and recognition in an age-dependent fashion in a very complex process.

In: Handedness: Theories, Genetics and Psychology ISBN: 978-1-61470-502-4
Editors: J. Dunham and T. Davenport

Chapter I

The Significance of Knot-tying Habits in Handedness Research and Forensic Science

Robert Chisnall
Faculty of Education, Queen's University, Kingston, Ontario, Canada

Abstract

Questionnaires, skill assessments – such as the Edinburgh and Briggs-Nebes Handedness Inventories – association analysis, brain scans, and other methods have been instrumental in a variety of research interests. A range of uni-manual preferences have been identified. Handedness, popularly assessed according to writing preferences, is not binary or one-dimensional. Evolving from Piaget's early work and epistemology, as well as traditional and experiential knotting acumen, the analysis of innate knot-tying habits is an esoteric field concerned with class-characteristic evidence in forensic science. Most relevant, focussed empirical investigations have yielded an analogous spectrum of preferences in one-wend and two-wend tying tasks – from the dominance of the more prevalent S enantiomers, which are strongly associated with dextrality, to the opposite or Z chiral form. Data and theoretical models linking handedness and tying habits are discussed, along with speculations regarding the potential in profiling tying habits and the importance of noting knot chirality in future research.

Introduction

For years the link between hand dominance and fundamental knot-tying habits has been intuited in crime scene identification and forensic science, and even in fictional accounts of criminal investigations, but the actual relationship only recently has undergone the scrutiny of peer-reviewed research. An understanding of the underlying mechanisms is starting to emerge, and this insight may be of benefit to handedness researchers as well as forensic investigators.

Herein, the relationship between hand dominance and tying habits will be examined. Initially, the discussion of handedness theories will range from anthropological and historical perspectives to genetic and neuroscience models. An examination of the challenges associated with defining and measuring handedness will follow. A survey of applicable knotting lore, assumptions, and esoteric terms and concepts will precede a review of research pertaining specifically to knot-tying behaviour. The relevance to forensic science of recent qualitative and quantitative investigations into tying habits will be outlined, and speculations regarding future research applications in psychology and related fields will be presented.

Some Preliminaries: Knot Nomenclature and Concepts

In order to discuss knot-tying research within the framework of handedness and laterality research, several essential concepts and terms must be clearly defined: tying landmarks, types of knots, knot capsizement or deformation, fundamental knot structures, and knot chirality (Ashley, 1944; Chisnall, 2000). Although the literature differs regarding standardization of knot names, herein all knot names will be capitalized (Chisnall, 2007).

A rope or cord consists of a wend or working end, a bight, and a standing part or stand for short. The bight forms the knot proper and the stand is the unknotted portion of the material being tied. There are several general types of knots. Here are a few broad definitions:

- Knots or knot masses are devoid of loops or attachments to other objects. They can occur anywhere in a rope or cord. The simplest knots are the Trefoil or Overhand Knot (Figure 1), which has three crossing points, and the Figure Eight Knot (Figure 2) and Pretzel Knot (Figure 3), which have four crossing points. (If there are any less than three crossing points, there is no structurally stable knot. With more crossings, the structure potentially becomes more complex.)

- Loops or loop knots may be fixed or 'slippery' (i.e., adjustable), and they may contain one or more loops. Overhand Loops and Overhand Slip Loops are illustrated in Figures 4 and 5.
- Bends join rope or cord wends. The simplest bends are parcelling or packaging knots called Granny Knots (Figure 6) and Reef Knots (Figure 7), the latter of which are sometimes called Square or Hercules Knots. Granny Knots, or Grannies, and Reefs each contain two Half Knots (Figure 8).
- Hitches attach ropes and cords to other objects and should not be confused with loops or loop knots. Hitches fall apart when removed from the object to which they are attached, while loops retain their structure. Simple Half Hitches are depicted in Figure 9.

Knots can capsize, flip over or deform into other structures – either accidentally of through deliberate action. For example, with some coaxing, the Figure Eight Knot can be deformed into a Pretzel Knot. When loaded asymmetrically, Granny Knots can change into Clove Hitches (Figure 10), and the Reef Knot can capsize into Girth Hitch (Figure 11). This is an important consideration when considering how a deformed knot may have been tied initially.

The most basic knot formations – which are of relevance to this discussion – include structures that have already been mentioned: Overhand Knots, Half Knots, Half Hitches, Overhand Slip Loops, Overhand Loops, Clove Hitches and Girth Hitches. Overhands are topologically similar to Half Hitches and Half Knots, which can be combined to form more complex structures. As already mentioned, for example, pairs of Half Knots form Granny Knots and Reef Knots. Grannies contain identical Half Knots, Clove Hitches contain identical Half Hitches, Reefs comprise two opposite Half Knots, and Girth Hitches consist of two opposite Half Hitches.

The majority of people tie simple, unsophisticated knots such as these. Complex knots, requiring specialized training and experience, are tied comparatively rarely (Chisnall, 2007; 2010a; 2010b). The average knot-tier repeatedly uses the primary structures described, often in multiples to form more secure combinations. Sequences of three of more Half Hitches or Half Knots can appear in everyday tying and in forensic evidence (knotted ligatures).

Germane to this analysis if the fact that the Overhand Knot and its equivalent structures each have two opposite variants or mirror images. Pairs of mirror images are called enantiomers or enantiomorphs, drawing on terminology from the field of chemistry. These pairs are said to be chiral to or have chirality. (The Figure Eight – and its topological equivalent, the Pretzel Knot – is amphichiral because it does not have a mirror image.) As mentioned, basic knots can be combined to form more complex structures. Grannies have equal enantiomers, while Reefs contain one of each chiral form, and these formations appear frequently.

Based on conventions used in textiles industries, anthropological terminology and evolving standards in forensic science, knot enantiomers are labelled S and Z, as illustrated (Canadian General Standards Board, 1984; Canadian Government Specifications Board, 1978; Wendrick, 1996; Chisnall, 2000). The S and Z designations are simple and unambiguous, and the fundamental shapes of these capital letters mimic the essential structures of the knots they label – specifically the crossing points. If the wraps or crossing points of a Trefoil are held vertically, as depicted n Figure 1, the distinguishing structures are obvious. The outer part of the Overhand Knot labelled S wraps up and to left, while the Z enantiomorph wraps up and to the right. Alternative but less-prevalent labelling systems include the following (Chisnall, 2000; Ide, 2009):

- Right and Left
- Right-Hand or Handed and Left-Hand or Handed
- R and L or RH and LH
- Dextral and Sinistral
- D and L
- ‘d’ and ‘l’ or L and D (nomenclature used in Great Britain)
- Levorotatory and Dextrorotatory (from organic chemistry)
- Dexiotrop and Laeotrop (from classical topology)
- N and Z (which can be confused when rotated ninety degrees.)

The S and Z nomenclature is widely accepted but not universal. Labelling a knot left-handed can introduce bias. Left-handed tiers do not consistently tie S or left-handed Overhand Knots. The S and Z designations have been established in the literature and they afford less ambiguity than other labelling systems such as the N or Z designations. The letters N and Z can be confused if these capital letters are turned sideways on any knot diagram employed to record anthropological findings or forensic evidence.

A number of these terms and concepts will be sporadically referenced in the historical review of the literature. They will certainly be critical when the research centring on knot-tying behaviour is examined later in detail. In particular, the S and Z enantiomorphs of these basic knot formations are significant to any enquiry related to handedness, and chirality should be noted carefully whenever tying tasks are integral to the research.

Manual Laterality: Historical Perspectives

Researchers have endeavoured to answer three fundamental questions:

- What is handedness?
- How can it be measured?
- What are its mechanisms?

These questions delve into the very nature of brain function and they have served to guide psychologists, educators, physicians, therapists, physiologists and other scientists in their quest to unravel numerous mysteries. What follows is a brief historical outline of theories that gave rise to current behavioural, genetic, and physiological models of laterality and handedness.

Anthropological and Historical Overview

Initial theories of handedness were sensitive to the statistical rarity of sinistrality. Modern theories are no different in that respect. However, early researchers concerned themselves with any historical or anthropological evidence that could be gleaned from a variety of sources, some of which have relevance to knot-tying habits.

It was thought that if consistent commonness of right-handedness could be determined, and roughly the same proportions occurred throughout all cultures and historical periods, then the underlying factor was biological. Conversely, if the proportion of dextrals and sinistrals could be shown to vary with social and technical changes, then handedness could be attributed to cultural influences. The classic nature-nurture controversy fuelled the philosophy and methodology of early research.

The questions investigators faced were simple but challenging. How could one determine the handedness of prehistoric people without written records? Even when written records were available, what evidence could be discerned? Answers were not obvious. Being less than rigidly empirical, the evidence unearthed seemed to create more indeterminacy than clarification.

Similarly, evidence of knot-tying habits in prehistoric societies was not immediate and obvious. Early use of knots and tying materials has been derived from secondary sources, such as preserved artifacts like amulets, since actual knotted animal and plant materials have long since decayed (Warner and Bednarik, 1996; Warner, 1996; Kleij, 1996).

Another approach was to examine the behaviour of modern primates and derive evolutionary and genetic arguments (Hopkins and Russell, 2004; Hopkins, et al. 2007). The manual laterality of spider monkeys has been studied (Laska, 1996), but knot-tying behaviour was not observed. Nest-making and knot-tying behaviour have been observed in wild gorillas and chimpanzees. There have been several reports of captive orangutans tying knots, as well, although close association with humans may have been an influential factor (Warner and Bednarik, 1996; Herzfeld and Lestel, 2006.). Seven orangutans, three bonobos and two chimpanzees, all of which were reared by humans and highly acculturated in zoos, were observed tying knots. Unfortunately, there is no indication in the literature of preferred S or Z enantiomers even though Half Hitches and Granny Knots were noted. Handedness relative to knot chirality has been ignored up to the present.

The literature variously reports that dextrality constitutes anywhere from 65% to 95% of the general human population (Michel and Harkins, 1985; Hannaford, 2005). Although, as Uomini (2009) reported, 85% of Homo sapiens are right-handed for most uni-manual actions, other great ape species do not display consistent laterlization. Evidence suggests that human dextrality may have emerged at the species level through the social transmission of increasingly complex tool use activities, wherein there is bimanual differentiation. There is clear evidence (Balter, 2009) from numerous Neanderthal skeletons that those prehistoric hominids tended to be right-handed. Detailed measurements of the dorsal inclination of the glenoid fossa, humeral length and head diameter, length and width, and radial and ulnar lengths can be used to determine handedness (Schulter-Ellis, 1980). Studies of human and nonhuman primates suggest that handedness varies in accordance with the complexity of the task and the skill level required to perform it (William, et al., 2007; Uonomi, 2009; Balter, 2009). Several studies have shown that manually challenging skills, such as knot-tying, are acquired more easily when the learners use the same left- and right-hand movements as their teachers. However, specific knot enantiomers were not recognized in this research and, therefore, could not be associated with tier handedness.

The indirect evidence of other Stone Age artifacts was ambiguous at times. The pattern of chipping on hand axes and tools showed that some were made by left-handers, others by right-handers (Silverstein and Silverstein, 1977). Cave paintings from Europe's Mammoth and Reindeer Periods gave further clues (Harris, 1980). A right-handed individual tends to draw figures and heads facing left when depicted in profile; left-handers find it easier to draw right-facing profiles (Silverstein and Silverstein, 1977). Both types of renderings were found in ancient paintings. Overall, the evidence was inconclusive and confusing. Prehistoric people were either ambidextrous or equally left- and right-handed.

There is agreement that right-handedness has predominated since the Old Testament (Harris, 1980). The Bible itself served as a source of evidence, although interpretations of the notable passages in Genesis, Psalms and Judges generated debate owing to differing translations. Tools and weapons acquired from the Bronze Age or later indicated the preeminence of the right hand (Silverstein and Silverstein, 1977). The Teta tomb at Gizeh (2,200 B.C.) houses stone carvings that show the right hand in an attitude of supplication. Bas-reliefs of ancient Assyrians and Cambodians highlighted the dominance of the right hand in wielding a sword (Harris, 1980). Many explanations were offered. It was speculated that a sword or spear held in an attacker's right-hand would have a better chance of piercing his enemy's leftward slanting heart, while the shield held in the left hand would better protect that more vulnerable side of the body (Silverstein and Silverstein, 1977). This was regarded as a weak theory because the slight leftward slant of the heart is actually insignificant. Evidence distilled from the artifacts and ruins of ancient Egyptians, Greeks, and Romans also lent credence to the notion that right-handedness was the norm during historical times (Silverstein and Silverstein, 1977; Wendrich, 1996). However, exact numbers could not be established. The determination of a constant and universal proportion in population handedness was impossible, and this was frustrating for researchers. To discover ambiguities and inconsistencies in the anthropological and historical evidence was to generate more unanswered questions. A simple choice between cultural and biological mechanisms could not be made (Harris, 1980). Theories combining physiological and societal explanations did develop though.

Early Theories

Early explanations of handedness can be divided into five main categories (Harris, 1980):

- those stressing structural asymmetries of the human body;
- theories linking handedness to cultural conditioning and learning;
- the search for hereditary mechanisms;
- speculations attributing handedness to a pathological state of brain or personality;
- and attributions of left-handedness to statistical rarity.

By modern standards, some of these approaches seem silly. It has taken years of careful research to dispel the prejudices and fallacies inherent in such notions, ideas that often hindered scientific inquiry or clouded emerging facts. However, some ideas were grounded in sound reasoning and they persist today as bases for more elaborate hypotheses.

Structural Asymmetry

Several prominent scientists of the 1800's suggested handedness could be explained by the asymmetrical arrangement of internal organs like the heart and liver. If these organs appeared as the mirror image of the normal visceral pattern, then the individual in question would be left-handed (Harris, 1980). With only vague clinical support, this theory became the subject of much discussion throughout European medical circles. It was all but forgotten eighty years later. However, visceral asymmetry remained a popular foundation for subsequent ideas.

Andrew Buchanan advanced a theory in 1862 that became well known (Beaton, 1985). He focussed on the asymmetry of the lungs and liver. The great weight of the liver was conjectured to cause a shift in balance to the left side, leaving the limbs on the right-hand side freer for action. Borelli and Weber used cadavers to make determinations regarding centre of balance, but nothing conclusive could be said about whether this point was situated in or displaced from the mesial plane relative to handedness (Harris, 1980; Netley, 1988). Several researchers of the period attempted to link this theory with embryology, but criticisms of visceral asymmetry as a theoretical base were frequent and harsh.

For several centuries, up until the 19th Century, certain blood-flow theories were pushed as explanations for handedness (Beaton, 1985). It was thought that differential blood flow to the arms was the cause of hand dominance. This idea, often called the 'subclavian theory' after the artery, did not survive when it was increasingly recognized in the 18th Century that the hemispheres of the brain and not the hands were the critical organs (Harris, 1980).

The work of Paul Broca (1827-1880) and anatomical characteristics of aphasic patients gave impetus to investigations of brain specialization. It was discovered that the third frontal convolution of the left hemisphere was the brain's centre of speech (Beaton, 1985). The discovery soon followed that the motor centre for a limb on one side of the body was in the opposite half of the brain. The notion of hemispheric dominance was born.

The brain attracted attention as a neurological basis for hand preference. Theories of handedness and brain dominance relied heavily on explanations stemming from physiological asymmetry: unequal blood supply to the halves of the brain, differential hemispheric weight, asymmetrical brain convolutions, and differences in fissure length. Each received varying degrees of acceptance and skepticism. Even though no firm explanation for handedness could be offered, the wheels were set in motion for future avenues of neurological and physiological research.

Pathological evidence in the mid-1800's indicated that there was a higher incidence of disease and deformity on the left side of the body (Harris, 1980; Beaton, 1985). This was viewed as additional support for the superiority of the right side of the body and emerging concepts of left hemispheric dominance. It also laid the ground work for pathological explanations of left-handedness.

The asymmetry of handedness was applied to other motor areas and all senses in the late 19th Century. The idea of ocular and auditory dominance contributed to the growing complexity of extant handedness theories. Despite the fact that no data could be generated to support a correlation between ocular and manual dominance, ocular dominance research persisted into the 20th Century.

The 'arm length' theory appeared in the literature in the 20th Century. It was proposed that student handedness could be determined by measuring the length of the ulna in both arms. The longer of the two indicated hand dominance. Psychologists and educators took notice (Harris, 1980). After numerous measurements, Beeley (1919) questioned whether this was a reliable indicator of handedness.

Despite the problems and misleading paths of inquiry, patently incorrect theories fell by the wayside while those bearing some basis in fact endured. Most significantly, the rudimentary ideas of neurophysiological asymmetry and brain dominance opened the doors to a rich and complex field of research (Steinmetz, et al., 1991; Jordan, Patching and Thomas, 2003; Sibner, et al., 2002; Sainburg, 2002; Sainburg and Schaefer, 2004).

Positional Asymmetry

A French physiologist named Joseph Achille Comte studied the birth positions in 20,539 cases (Harris, 1980). The data accumulated suggested some link to hand preference. He found that in 96% of birth presentations the vertex of the newborn's skull appeared first. Of these, 17,226 were reported to have first or left occipito-anterior positions (the infant's head facing the mother's right) while 2,153 involved second or 'right' position presentations (the infant's head facing left). Comte proposed that birth presentation was a clue to the infant's intrauterine position.

He was unable to prove, however, that newborns appearing in the first and second birth positions definitely became right-and left-handed respectively. For this reason the 'birth presentation' theory was overlooked, although it did reappear three more times under other authors. Ultimately, Overstreet (1938) concluded that there was no correlation between handedness and prenatal position.

The importance of uterine orientation reemerged relative to twins. It was found that there was a higher incidence of sinistrality among dizygotic and monozygotic twins (Wilson and Jones, 1932). Researchers were not willing to discuss a direct relationship between fetal position and handedness phenomena though. It was emphasized that such a relationship deserved consideration and that attitude remained (Harris, 1980; Beaton, 1985).

Pathological Left-Handedness

Accepting any one of the physiological or social theories discussed already, many scientists went one step further to say that left-handedness was a manifestation of some brain disorder, personality pathology, or both. These models tended to be most interesting to study and yet most unfair to left-handers because they focused on negative characteristics (Harris, 1980).

Sinistrality has been the target of negative cultural, educational, linguistic, and religious traditions. It is, therefore, no wonder that scientific theories eventually emerged which held left-handedness, as a state of degeneracy, accountable for the development of criminality and antisocial behaviour.

Geneticists viewed it as a recessive trait linked to aspects of diminished mental ability and moral excellence (Jordan, 1911).

In 1903, a noted Italian criminologist named Cesare Lombroso reported that the proportion of left-handers was higher among certain types of criminals than among soldiers (Beaton, 1985). An anatomical study of criminal heads led him to believe that normal individuals had greater development in their left hemisphere while the converse was true of criminals and deviants. Smith (1917) examined delinquents and children in American 'industrial schools' concluding that wickedness accompanies left-handedness. These conclusions were remarkable considering that the surveys of the time were unrepresentative (Harris, 1980).

Several early writers criticised this work, pointing out that left-handedness was not necessarily a stigma of inferiority. Two types of left-handedness were named (Satz, 1972): the atavistic or constitutional type was attributed to an inversion of normal cerebral asymmetry; the pathological kind manifested after a cerebral lesion, predominated in epileptics and delinquents (Jordon, 1911; Brewster, 1913). This classification system anticipated later thinking (Satz, 1972).

Burt, an educational psychologist, and Blau, a psychoanalyst, were very influential proponents of the pathological view. Left-handedness was associated with infantile psychoneurosis, stubbornness, disobedience, and insecurity. These theorists were undaunted by the fact that their clinical evidence did not support their contentions (Harris, 1980; Boake, et al., 1983; Beaton, 1985; Charlton, 1988).

Various cultures symbolically associate the left hand with feminine traits as well as evilness (Silverstein and Silverstein, 1977; Witelson and Pallie, 1973). This view was echoed in early anatomical writings, wherein left-handedness was linked with the female state and specific reproductive functions were thought to occur on the left side in the female body.

Even more extreme, left-handedness was regarded as an indicator of deviance and homosexuality in men (Barsley, 1966). Wilhelm Fliess, Sigmund Freud's closest friend outlined a theory of bisexuality which included bilateralism and left-handedness (Bonaparte, Freud, and Kris, 1954). Freud was interested in this notion, but felt that any direct association between sexual disturbance and criminality was doubtful and inapplicable. Considering the strange relationship Freud and Fliess had, it is difficult to imagine that they were capable of objective inquiry regarding this area of research.

Once left-handedness had been linked to homosexuality, it did not take long before emotional, artistic, and sensitive characteristics were associated with sinistrality. Considerable mention was made of Leonardo da Vinci and

Michelangelo, both of whom were left-handed (Silverstein and Silverstein, 1977; Harris, 1980).

The attribution of cognitive deficiencies soon followed. Stuttering and reversed writing were reported to occur more frequently among sinistral individuals. This soon led to the idea that the motor centres for writing and speaking were intimately associated with the language centre in the human brain (Beaton, 1985). It was thought that natural left-handers, when forced to write with the right, could develop problems in speech and writing habits, including dyscriptia, dysgraphia and dyslexia. Reversal of hand use, accordingly, was believed to relieve stuttering. A link between language and handedness was made, and work in this area continues

It was also believed that left-handers were deficient in spatial cognitive abilities, owing to the incidence of mirror writing and so forth. Again, Leonardo's famous mirror writing style was often cited (Silverstein and Silverstein, 1977; Harris, 1980). It was thought that mirror writing was a natural method for sinistrals because they would tend to write from right to left. Detractors of the theory that left-handers are deficient in spatial cognition and intelligence often cited Lewis Carroll, another left-hander, and Leonardo as examples to the contrary.

Despite all of the very damaging notions that developed over the years, some useful ideas emerged and into the research pathology of handedness continues (Michael, et al., 2005). Even though the question of forcing left-handers to write with their right persisted until the 1950's, more psychologists and pediatricians came to agree that coercion was ineffective and dangerous in education. Finally, the prejudices of sexuality and temperament dissipated under a wave of objective inquiry and clinical research throughout the medical, psychological and educational fields (Beaton, 1985; Harris, 1980).

Cultural Conditioning

It was as early as the 17th Century when 'nurturists' started rallying against the 'nativists' regarding the theoretical basis of hand preference. They were convinced that handedness did not depend on heredity or physiological asymmetries. Rather, they believed dextral predominance was strictly the result of learning and societal conditioning. Elements of their theories described below have lingered to this day.

In the 1880s, the importance of the child's position while being nursed or carried by the mother was held to have an influence on hand preference (Harris,

1980; Beaton, 1985). It was conjectured that, in most instances, a nurse would carry a child on her right arm, thus leaving the infant's right arm free to move and develop. The infant-holding theory had one immediate problem though. It was observed that mothers commonly carry their children in the left arm. This was confirmed by Burt (1937) through personal observation of 100 mothers, as well as a survey of artistic depictions of the Madonna and Child.

The warfare-shield theory, as described earlier, pointed to historical evidence that indicated dextrality was the norm because the heart side of the body needed protection. Critics of this theory cited the use of single-handed implements like the club and javelin. Shields were not employed with these weapons. Cultural one-handedness would have developed long before the advent of the shield, and another point emerged. If left-handers were more vulnerable by failing to protect the left their bodies, why did they survive (Silverstein and Silverstein, 1977; Harris, 1980)?

These theories received little attention in the 19th Century. Nurturists focussed on the actual hand preference of the human infant. Studies of babies and children were undertaken as sources of critical information both for and against the societal-conditioning view of handedness. Several researchers presented observations of their own children but drew no conclusions (Harris, 1980). The first truly experimental investigation was performed by James Baldwin (1890; 1894) using his daughter as a subject. He elicited unsymmetrical reaching behaviour by presenting objects just beyond her grasp. From the results, he concluded that his daughter had developed right-handedness under the pressure of muscular effort.

Similar investigations by others followed 15 years later. Their conclusions supported the premise that right-handedness was a normal part of physiological development, not a phenomenon controlled by training (Nice, 1918; Woolley, 1910).

These theories depended fundamentally on some sort of physiological explanation of handedness. However, in the 1920s the American scientific community shifted toward behaviourism under the influence of John Watson (Beaton,1985). His research showed no uniformity in hand use nor fixed differentiation of response in either hand until a societal influence impinged upon an individual's behaviour. Watson was at a loss to explain how society could have consisted of a predominantly right-handed population to begin with. The existence of sinistrals could not be accounted for as well.

Despite deficiencies in these behavioural and developmental theories, the effects of societal convention and learning were known to hold some importance in the development of individual handedness. It was becoming apparent that handedness was not a simple phenomenon. Several factors, including heredity, conditioning, and physiology, were contributing to each person's hand preference. The mechanism was simply not one-dimensional.

At the turn of the 20th Century, there was a movement afoot that disputed the naturalness of dextral preferences. It was proposed that ambidexterity could ensue from rational education which allowed or encouraged individuals to develop naturally (Harris, 1980). This curious educational movement promised equal acquisition of writing and other skills by both hands. One proponent even went so far as to claim that both hands could carry out separate tasks independently because the brain, having two hemispheres, could be regarded as a 'double organ', one capable of accommodating separate and distinct thinking processes simultaneously (Jackson, 1905).

The most dramatic claim made concerning the benefit of ambidextral training was the promise that the effects of unilateral brain injury would be prevented or ameliorated by two-handed training (Harris, 1980).

The biggest criticism of the ambidextral culture was its apparent disregard for all of the accumulated evidence showing handedness to be innate and rooted in brain physiology (Crichton-Browne, 1907). This movement eventually subsided, falling victim to its own exaggerated claims and the preponderance of many other criticisms. However, some later educators continued to promote the benefits of two-handedness that had been promised earlier (Harris, 1980).

Hand Posture in Writing

Of any asymmetrical activity undertaken in our society today, handwriting is used most frequently to distinguish sinistrals from dextrals because it is simple and obvious (Barsley, 1970). The attention paid to writing habits by psychologists stems from the classical traditions of education, the teaching of penmanship the right-handed way (Beaton, 1985). Now, fortunately, students may develop the writing hand of their choice without disciplinary repercussions. Aside from the obvious humanistic and educational benefits of this trend, there have been research benefits. Another clue to the mystery of lateralization in the brain has been revealed – this being hand posture, particularly in the writing habits of sinistrals.

Individuals not only differ in their choice of writing hand but also in writing posture. Some utilize the normal position, in which the hand and forearm are kept straight, while others use the hooked or inverted position, in which the wrist is kept bent (Beaton, 1985).

It was suggested that the hooked position in left-handers prevented smudged writing and allowed the writer to see more clearly what was being written. With this argument, it was predicted that there would be a higher incidence of hooked dextral Israeli writers than Americans because Hebrew script proceeds from right to left (Herron, 1980). A greater frequency of Israeli dextrals with the inverted hand posture was not found, but it was also discovered that the inverted left-hander was less abundant among Israeli writers than among Americans (Shanon, 1978). A cultural or learning effect was suggested. As well, recent investigations have indicated that the inverted writing posture is more common among males than among females (Coren and Porac, 1979), thus suggesting a genetic or physiological mechanism.

It is generally understood that motor control in the upper limbs is performed by the contralateral hemisphere. There is evidence indicating this is true for the fine movements carried out by the distal musculature of the fingers (Herron, 1980; Beaton, 1985). It has been suggested that hand posture can reveal what part of the brain is controlling an individual's writing actions.

Levy and Reid (1976) proposed that upright or normal handwriting postures indicate there is contralateral hemispheric control for language in its written forms. Conversely, inverted hand postures were deemed to signify ipsilateral cerebral control. Some controversy over this hypothesis was generated by physiological research into neural pathways.

Moscovitch and Smith (1979) interpreted the results of their research as indicating that the inverted and normal writing postures could be attributed to differences in visuo-motor rather than sensori-motor organization. However, there is ample evidence throughout the literature pointing

out differences in fine-motor or sensori-motor control as an explanation for writing postures (Barsley, 1970; Herron, 1980; Parlow, 1978; Beaton, 1985), and throughout this research it generally has been found that, unlike dextrals, sinistrals with normal writing postures show an advantage for the right hand in finger flexion. This suggests that the differences in writing posture can be explained by sensori-motor organisation as originally hypothesized by Levy and Reid (1976).

Considering the complexity of the human brain, it may be discovered in future research that visuo-motor and sensori-motor factors are intricately organized in the determination of hand preference and writing control. Other more subtle elements may be discovered as well.

Genetics and Heredity versus Environmental Theories

At the turn of the 20th Century, speculation regarding the genetic basis of handedness took root (Beeley, 1919; Harris, 1980). Even Darwin had addressed this issue using his own child as a case study. German researchers were the strongest proponents while others explicitly denied any link to genetics whatsoever.

Very few systematic genetic investigations were performed in those early years and the results were often unclear. Subsequent family surveys produced clearer results. Of particular note, numerous double left-handed matings giving rise to entire families of sinistral offspring were recorded.

In 1922, Jordan wrote with assurance that left handedness was clearly genetic, and that the incidence of sinistrality closely followed the rules of inheritance as they were understood at that time. Several others supported this view (Ramaley, 1913), but a strictly recessive model predicted that left-handed couples would always produce left-handed children, and this was not the case. Recognition of learning effects and a growing awareness of the complexity of genetic mechanisms presaged further investigation and controversy. The genetic mystery would not be solved by a simple dominant-recessive model.

Still, reports of left-handed families were compiled. In one remarkable case, two left-handed parents produced children, all preferring the left hand (Harris, 1980). Some family surveys had weak report reliability. Nevertheless, a genetic influence was definitely indicated even though the underlying system was not yet clear. There were also suggestions that the defining of handedness was not a straightforward undertaking. Assumption of a strictly dichotomous classification system was deemed to be possibly misleading (Beaton, 1985).

Even in the 1970s and 1980s the inheritance of handedness was disputed (Corballis, 1980). Levy and Nagylaki (1972) proposed a model that explained variations in handedness and cerebral lateralization in terms of Mendelian principles. This view was founded on a tradition of genetic models occupying most of the 20th Century. Such investigators as Trankell (1955), Rife (1940), and Ramaley (1913) were just three who held firmly to the position that handedness was solely attributable to heredity. They disregarded the accumulating evidence which suggested a learning effect.

The environmental position has been hotly contended as well (Collins, 1988). Dextrality was regarded as a learned response to a right-handed environmental bias. Hence, left-handedness was deemed a failure to learn, either through physical defect, faulty education, or 'emotional negativism.' This, essentially, had been the nurture side of the argument. One can quickly identify notions that resemble the dangerous and prejudiced ideas of earlier research. Despite these extreme views, it is generally held that there is a genetic influence (Corballis, 1980; Beaton, 1985).

Annett (1972) proposed a model that is a compromise between these opposing views and was generally regarded as the more plausible genetic explanation (Corballis, 1980). Two fundamental suppositions were made. First, unsystematic environmental influences are the cause of a large random component in the distribution of inter-manual differences. Second, most people inherit a 'right shift' factor, perhaps through a single gene, such that the mean distribution favours dextrality. Some people may lack this gene. Annett further conjectured that these individuals should favour either hand equally on unbiased tests. Proof was later furnished that the lack of a right shift is a recessive trait (Annett, 1974).

Subsequent research found fault with Annett's model and data, but it is widely accepted that a genetic factor may well explain the overall bias among humans toward right-handedness and the left-cerebral control of speech (Corballis, 1980). In answer to criticisms of previous work, Annett (1978) indicated that accidental variation is likely a major determinant of handedness, and dextral bias is induced by a genetic factor.

The underlying genetic mechanisms are more complex. Current disagreement concerns the cause of left-handedness. Although Annett argued that some incidence of sinistrality could be explained in terms of a recessive trait, many believe there is insufficient evidence to support this notion (Corballis, 1980; Beaton, 1985). Many researchers held that environmental causes are at the root of sinistrality, but this notion garnered decreasing attention. According to Carter-Saltzman (1980), the results of a shared biological heritage, rather than sociological factors, are more significant in hand preference.

More recent research revealed that the LRRTM1 gene appears to play a key role in determining which parts of the brain control specific functions, including the flip to left-handedness (Francks, at el., 2007).

Developmental Psychology and Learning Implications

The scientific dispute over whether handedness is a genetic, physiological, or environmental phenomenon continued. However, many of the old fallacies fell under a growing legacy of reliable and convincing research data.

It is now known that dextrality has some genetic basis while societal and environmental pressures influence left-handedness through learning effects. Currently, investigators recognize that gross-motor, upper-limb movements are contralaterally controlled. The neurological pathways for fine-motor or sensori-motor movements are being unravelled. Research supports the theory that the speech centres in the brain can be associated with the motor centres that control the dominant hand. It is known that there is a higher occurrence of sinistrals among twins and males in the human population. Credence is also given to the opinion that left-handedness can be a response to pathological factors in some cases. Important questions still remain unanswered.

Beyond the constructs of psychology and the mechanisms of genetics and physiology, handedness exists as a holistic phenomenon. It is a unique expression of an individual's connection to his or her environment and it has social and pedagogical implications.

Piaget contributed considerably to the understanding of spatial-visual relationships in the cognitive development of children. In particular, he examined how the developing mind deals with the relativistic spatial notions of 'neighbourhood,' 'between' and 'surrounding' (Piaget, 1951; 1977; Piaget and Inhelder, 1967; Olson, 1970; Eliot and Salking, 1975). Strohecker (1989a, 1989b, 1989c, 1990, 1991, 1996) further explored older children's ideas about creating and classifying knots, as well as their development of topological concepts, and Caron-Pargue (1983, 1985) explored how verbal and graphical encoding of knot forms are related.

As Tichy and Belacek (2009) and other researchers (Ramsay, 1980) discovered, handedness manifests in infants between seven and 13 months of age, and it is well established in 3-year-old children. Laterality appears to be stabilized by year ten. An investigation of the degree of correlation between handedness and physiological neocebellar extinction syndrome, confirmed that the motor cortex of the left hemisphere, in connection with the right cerebellar hemisphere, is responsible for cerebellar dominance and handedness. There has been evidence that handedness develops in the womb (Hepper and Shahidullah, 1990; 1991; Hepper, et al., 1998). Laterality, which appears to be stabilized in children by the age of 10, "appears to be a structurally arranged complex of physiological phenomena not quite dependent on one another" (Tichy and Belacek, 2009, p. 18). Data pertaining to cross-footedness indicated that neocerebral dominance correlates with hand dominance, which suggests that the learning of new asymmetrical or uni-manual skills – such as the tying of sophisticated knots – will be governed by established hand dominance and brain laterality.

This, and similar research, provides a foundation for why it has been long understood that early forced learning relative to preferred handedness can have detrimental effects on an individual student's speech, reading and writing (Beaton, 1985; Clark, 1974). There may be other negative outcomes. This holds particular significance for modern educators, especially those concerned with language arts, and probably instructors of physical education and outdoor recreation (Clark, 1974; Grady, 1984).

How exactly learning and environmental influences interact with handedness to produce observable tying habits is unclear. However, research data shed some light on this question.

Michel and Harkins (1985) examined how the concordance of handedness between teacher and students can facilitate learning manual skills. It was found that, "Learning was greatly facilitated by concordance of handedness between teacher and student." and the researchers conjectured that, ". . . it is conceivable that observational learning of manual skill, which accompanied hominid evolution of tool-use and tool-making skills, could have provided selective pressure for concordance (the right-bias) in human handedness." (p. 597). Participants were asked to tie three knots: the Sheepshank (Figure 12), a "mountain climbing non-slip knot" (likely the Alpine Butterfly; Figure 13), and a "magic slip-knot" (p. 598). These knots were not depicted, their chirality and variations were not indicated, the detailed methods of knot instruction were not described, and the exact configuration of the magic slip-knot was not specified. It may have been a conventional Overhand Slip Knot (Figure 5) or a Figure Eight Slip Knot (Figure 13), for example. In light of research pertaining to knot-tying behaviour (Chisnall, 2009; 2010a; 2011), which will be described later, the exact configuration of each knot tied, along with the chirality of the component structures, could be important to a complete understanding of teacher-learner concordance relative to handedness.

Neurological, Molecular and Brain-Scan Research

In 2003, Tracy, et al. reported the results of an investigation that involved knot-tying tasks and brain imaging techniques. Subjects were trained to tie relatively complex knots. Functional Magnetic Resonance Imaging (fMRI) was used to discover that subjects who learned the task well exhibited new regional brain activity in posterior and medial structures, like the posterior spatial gyrus. The Edinburgh Handedness Inventory determined that all 15 subjects were strongly right-handed, and subjects were taught to tie a Sheep Shank (Figure 12) and a Sheet Bend (Figure 14), according to the figures provided in that paper. Their findings were summarized as follows (p. 904): "The new activation for the pattern of strong learning has alternative interpretations involving whither retrieval during episodic memory of a shift toward non-executive cognitive control of the task. While these interpretations are not resolved, the study makes clear that single time-point images of motor skill can be misleading because the brain structures that implement action can change following practice."

It should be noted that the Sheep Shank, having two component Half Hitches that are chiral, has four variants. An S/Z or Z/S configuration (depending on the order of tying) was illustrated in the paper cited. Similarly, there are four basic forms of the Sheet Bend, although the direct S[1] version was depicted. However, there was no discussion of the influence that knot chirality may have on learning and performance relative to tier handedness. Which particular enantiomers are demonstrated or depicted, and how they are presented, might have an effect.

Leff, et al. (2006) reported on the feasibility of Near Infrared Spectroscopy (NIRS) for studying subjects performing realistic knot-tying surgical tasks. A recognisable haemodynamic response to brain activation was observed, and this was reliable and repeatable. They concluded that (p. 141): "A wide range of prefrontal activation was observed, thought to reflect considerable variation in the cognitive resources allocated to complete an attention-demanding surgical task [knot-tying]." A follow-up study (Leff, et al., 2008) produced data suggesting prefrontal processing is affected by experience. Prefrontal activation is associated with technical performance adaptation in novices. Once again, the knots and their respective chiralities were not specified. Although these studies utilized knot-tying tasks, the possible interplay between knot chirality and uni-manual performance was ignored.

Other brain research has concentrated on handedness and uni-manual or lateralized skills other than knot-tying. For example Siebner, et al. (2002), in a positron emission tomography study on handwriting in converted left-handers, found that innate right-handers show a predominantly left-hemispheric activation of parietal and premotor association areas, whereas converted left-handers demonstrated a more bilateral activation pattern, with distinct activation in the right hemisphere, which may indicate suppression of unwanted left-hand movements.

The puzzle of brain asymmetry and handedness has been considered at the molecular level as well (Tao and Alsh, 2006). As more sophisticated means of brain analysis come to bear, the neurological underpinnings of brain laterality and handedness, amongst other physiological asymmetries, will be investigated and

[1] Sheet Bends can have an S or 'b' structure. The S indicates the chirality of the Overhand Slip Loop into which an S Sheet Bend can capsize. The 'b' indicates the shape of that portion of the Sheet Bend's internal structure that self-crosses. Z Sheet Bends can distort into Z Overhand Slip Loops, and they have a 'd'-shaped crossing-point structure. See Figure 13.

understood in greater detail. If knot-tying tasks are employed, hopefully chirality relative to handedness will be taken into account.

Recent Research

As noted, scientists from a wide range of disciplines – notably psychology, psychiatry, neurology, anatomy, and biology – have been investigating laterality differences in humans, and other species. Researchers in education have devoted some effort to the question of handedness. Sociology, anthropology, primate research, and comparative anatomy studies also contributed to evolving perspectives. Over the last half century, many studies on this subject have been published, only a few of which have been briefly described herein.

Current theories have been built upon the sounder ideas that have endured from early investigations and speculation. Considering the complexity of the human brain, it may be discovered in future research that visuo-motor and sensori-motor factors are intricately organized in the determination of hand preference, skill and writing control. Other more subtle elements may be discovered as well.

The scientific discussion pertaining to genetic, physiological, and environmental factors will continue, and old fallacies have fallen under a legacy of reliable and convincing research data. It is now known that dextrality has a neuroanatomical and genetic basis while societal and environmental pressures influence handedness through learning effects.

Beyond the constructs of psychology and the mechanisms of genetics and physiology, handedness exists as a holistic phenomenon. It is a unique expression of an individual's connection to his or her environment and it has social and pedagogical implications. The challenge for investigators has been and will continue to be associated with how to assess handedness.

The Challenge of Measuring Handedness

It can be a misleading oversimplification to determine whether one hand is superior over another based on individual respondents. Handedness is more complex than a simple binary attribution. The relationship of the right hand to the left depends on how the various digits are coordinated to execute different tasks in a finely programmed sequence of movements, and both hands can share complex tasks in varying ways (Herron, 1980; Beaton, 1985).

There are two fundamental questions faced by researchers. How should handedness be defined? How can it be reliably measured? This determination has been quite often arbitrary, which accounts for many of the contradictions throughout the handedness literature (Provins, 1967; Oldfield, 1971; Todor and Doane, 1977; Annett et al., 1979; Ransil and Schacter, 1994; Dragovic and Hammond, 2007), especially prior to 2000. Historically, people have been classified into three basic types: dextral, sinistral, and ambidextral – and more recently the terms mixed, inconsistent or shared handedness have been employed (Provins, 1967; Miller, 1971; Flowers, 1975, 1983; Steingruber, 1975; Briggs and Nebes, 1975; Bryden, 1977; Peters and Durding, 1978; Loo and Schneider, 1979; Peters, 1981). This simple classification does not account for the full range of manual asymmetry which can be observed. Handedness is more realistically modelled as a continuous distribution ranging from strongly right-handed to strongly left-handed (Annett, 1970; 1992; Peters and Durding,1978).

There are two distinguishable aspects of handedness that must be recognized in surveys: preference and skill. Numerous traditional techniques dominate this research. The Edinburgh Handedness Inventory has been employed extensively (Oldfield, 1971). Annett (1967) utilized a questionnaire that distinguished 12 behaviours or tasks. After analysing the responses from 2,321 subjects, Annett determined that there are at least 23 types of hand preference. It was then argued that handedness should not be regarded as a discrete variable. This inquiry was followed up using a peg-moving task (Annett, 1970). It was found that the degree of preference, as assessed by a questionnaire, correlated with the times taken by the two hands to place pegs into close-fitting holes. Conversely, Todor and Doane (1977) found a diminishing degree of correlation between left-handed manual preference and the difference in left-hand proficiency scores as task difficulty increased. However, it has been argued that the latter investigation produced a somewhat misleading conclusion (Beaton, 1985). By increasing task difficulty, the nature of the task is altered, and there is no reason to suppose that there is the same degree of symmetry between the hands regarding different components of movement control.

Using the Annett Hand Preference Questionnaire, Dragovic and Hammond (2007) found that 66% of those surveyed were consistently right-handed, 9.8% were consistently left-handed, 24.2% indicated inconsistent or mixed handedness. It was recommended that this questionnaire be updated with modern or relevant tasks. Other survey instruments and external methods of assessing brain laterality and uni-manual dexterity have included the Briggs-Nebes modified version of Annett's Handedness Inventory (Briggs and Nebes, 1975; Loo and Schneider, 1979), the Purdue Pegboard test of manual dexterity in conjunction with the

Edinburgh Handedness Inventory (Verdino and Dingman, 1998), Bishop's reaching card test (Doyen and Carlier, 2002), and a multivariate approach using hand preference and hand performance measures (Annett, 1992; Corey and Hurley, 2001; Brown, et al., 2006)). The notion of continuously distributed handedness is widely accepted.

The assumption that laterality should be evaluated along a unidimensional continuum was later brought into question (Corey and Hurley, 2001). A lattice analysis was employed to determine if the structure of hand preference was equal for dextrals and sinistrals. Within the limits of a small sample space, right-handed behaviour appeared to be more global while nearly all left-handers exhibited distinct profiles.

Calvert (1998) discovered that, when performing an unskilled motor task, left-handers showed greater readiness to use the non-preferred hand than right-handers. Similarly, Crovitz and Zener (1962) reported that left-handers are less consistently sinistral in their manual preference than right-handers are dextral. This is a problem when classifying left- and right-handed groups. Bryden (1977) found that dextrals show a strong preference for the right hand when tested objectively, but many who describe themselves as left-handed will in fact preferentially use the right hand for a number of activities. Left-handers vary more in their reporting of hand use than dextrals, and the within-subject consistency in hand use for particular tasks among sinistrals is also lower. This pointed out that the criteria for surveying left-handers should be more universal and better defined. Calvert (1998), employing a behavioural continuum, found that left-handers showed greater readiness to use the non-preferred hand than right-handers when performing an unskilled task.

Two types of movement were distinguished by Flowers in 1975. 'Ballistic' hand movements are made without feedback (like throwing a ball) while 'corrective' motions require a feedback loop to monitor and modify hand motions (like carrying a spoon of soup up to the mouth, or tying a knot). It was found that in strongly lateralized individuals – either dextrals or sinistrals – the preferred hand performed better than the non-preferred hand when it came to corrective movements. 'Ambilateral' or ambidextrous individuals showed poor control in the preferred hand without any compensatory increase in the skill of the non-preferred hand. Flowers (1975, 1983) also found that individuals having a manual preference that was not so distinct showed superior skill in the non-preferred hand. Hence, hand skill depends on the degree of manual preference and whether the required task is ballistic or corrective. Further, Steehuis and Bryden (1989) identified four types of handedness: skilled actions, reaching actions, power actions and bimanual actions. Knot-tying would seem to fit best into the later category.

Hand differences also depend upon the type of movement and its complexity (Steingruber, 1975; Provins, 1967; Peters, 1981). Practice seems to diminish the difference in skill level between the hands for certain tasks while the asymmetry remains constant for others. This was investigated by Annett, Hudson and Turner in 1979. It was found that the non-preferred hand was slower and more variable during the aiming phases of tasks (corrective movements).

Nakamura and Saito (1974) recorded electrical measurements of muscle contractions. Reaction times were faster for the preferred hand in supination but the non-preferred hand was quicker in flexion. This led them to believe that the two movements are controlled separately in the brain. It has been found that flexion of digits was carried out more quickly and with greater precision by left-hand fingers in people preferring the right hand (Kimura and Vanderwolf, 1970; Parlow, 1978). The relationship between the individual fingers is quite subtle and this further complicates the determination of skill differences between the right and left hands.

Hence, investigators are faced with the task of measuring handedness by degrees through examinations of hand skill and preference as separate characteristics. Types of skill, like corrective and ballistic, must be distinguished. The aim is to render more reliable conclusions by applying universal definitions and criterion cutoffs to data acquired through questionnaires and direct observations.

Investigations of Knot-Tying Habits

When it comes to knot-tying tasks, it can be speculated that the link between hand preference and skill may be substantial. Tiers surely will rely on the most efficient hand sequence that provides successful results. As previous research indicates, there are degrees of handedness, a spectrum of variability from dextrality to sinistrality. As the following discussion illustrates, examinations of the simplest knot-tying habits have revealed that there is a similar or parallel spectrum, wherein tiers prefer one of the two basic mirror-image knot structures: S and Z.

The question then becomes, to what extent do these two spectra correlate? Is one particular tying habit associated more strongly with left- or right-handedness?

Does the pattern of gradation between left- and right-hand dominance parallel the gradation from one basic knot structure to its mirror image?

There are indications that basic tying habits are innate – and to some extent 'lateralized' in that one enantiomer is preferred over the other, and one hand probably dominates in elementary tying tasks – while sophisticated knot-tying skill derived from training and experience could influence basic tying habits and vice versa.

Researching Knot-Tying Behaviour

The literature in psychology and epistemology refers to knot-tying relative to learning and cognition (Piaget, 1951; 1977; Piaget and Inhelder, 1967; Caron-Pargue , 1983; 1985; Strohecker, 1990; 1991). However, there has been very little written about knot-tying, knot chirality and handedness (Chisnall, 2000: 2007). At the outset three studies of any significance addressed tier habit and handedness, and these were comparatively informal investigations conducted by individuals with practical interests in knots: Des Pawson (1992), Dale Nute and Richard Haas (Budworth, 1985). This was followed by some peer-reviewed research in more recent years.

Geoffrey Budworth, a founding member of the International Guild of Knot Tyers, outlined the results of two investigations in *Knots and Crime* (1985). Both focussed on tier handedness, knotting knowledge, and tying consistency.

A "controlled experiment" (Budworth, 1985, p. 43) was conducted by Richard Haas involving approximately 40 subjects. About 50% of the right-handers tied S/S Grannies, and approximately 50% of left-handers produced Z/Z Grannies (Figure 6). Hence, these results suggested there is no correlation between handedness and knot chirality.

Subsequently, a "controlled experiment with approximately 40 individuals" was conducted by Richard Haas, an Investigator with the District Attorney's Office Bureau of Investigation in Ventura, California (Budworth, 1985, p. 43). No methodological details were reported other than the fact that some of the subjects were dextral and some were sinistral. The results are stated as follows: "About 50% of the [right-handed] people tied a [left-hand] Granny Knot. About the same percentage of [left-handers] tied a [right-hand] Granny Knot." (Budworth, 1985, p. 43).

A second study was performed by Dale H. Nute (1986), a member of the International Guild of Knot Tyers. Each of 103 college students was given a short length of cord and asked to tie a knot as if he or she were tying someone up.

Nute's aim was to determine the frequency one might expect to find in the general population of left-handed, LH, S, or S-twisting knots and hitches as well as right-handed, RH, Z, or Z-twisting knots and hitches. He also wanted some indication of the variety and frequency of knots people tie.

Of the 103 college students surveyed, 40% of the students tied Granny Knots and 81% tied Overhand Knots or knots based on the Overhand Knot. Only seven out of the 103 subjects tied sophisticated knots, these being the Bowline, Stevedore's Knot, Hangman's Knot, and Fisherman's Knot (not illustrated). Three out of every four dextrals tied RH or Z-twisting hitches while five of the seven left-handers tied LH or S-twisting hitches. The latter results suggest that there may be some link between tier handedness and the preferred chirality. However, these results run contrary to data from all subsequent inquiries, and it has been suggested that there may have been a transcription error in the reporting – RH and LH somehow got transposed. This is merely a speculation.

Nute asked several of the students surveyed to tie knots over a period of four to five years. "All consistently reproduced the same form of knot" they had originally tied (i.e., S or Z hitches and knots) and "most had considerable difficulty in tying the opposite form when asked to do so." (Budworth, 1985, p.44). He also discovered that this force of habit in tying one particular enantiomer can be overridden when individuals tie knots in an awkward position, like behind their heads. Twenty out of 27 students changed the handedness of their Granny or Reef Knots when asked to tie them overhead Ten actually changed the knot itself from a Granny to a Reef or vice versa.

In the late 1970's, Ron Underwood investigated a multiple murder at Farham in England. Underwood, who retired in 1983 as the Detective Chief Superintendent in Surrey, discovered that three young children and their mother had been strangled with nylon stockings. There was evidence to indicate that the mother had murdered her children and then committed suicide. However, the chirality of the knots used to tie the ligatures around the necks of the children was opposite to that of the hitches securing the stocking around the mother's neck (Underwood, 1988). An explanation was required, so eight police women were asked to tie stockings around their necks and around pieces of wood. He found that all eight reversed the twist of the hitches when tying nylons around their own necks, which concurs with Nute's findings.

According to Budworth (1985), habits are difficult to break. Individual skills persist under stress. In Nute's study, subjects found it difficult to reverse the handedness of their knots. Therefore, one could expect that volunteer subjects would not deliberately and easily alter their normal tying habits during a behavioural investigation.

Some years later, Des Pawson (1992) revisited this question. Sixty-three subjects were asked to tie Overhand Knots and Reef Knots. They produced a total of 70 knot samples. Most of the subjects had prior knotting experience or training. The results suggested that right-handers tend to prefer S-twisting Overhand Knots while there was an insufficient number of left-handers to make any conclusions. It also appeared that the right-handers sampled prefer the S/Z version of the Reef Knot. To what extent do these results indicate latent habits, and to what extent do they reveal previous learning and experience?

In 1985, as a precursor to a more formal and lengthy inquiry, a preliminary investigation of knot tying habits was conducted (Chisnall, 1994; 2000; 2010). Twenty-four subjects were involved, six females and 18 males. Each subject was asked to tie a piece of cord around a spar and secure it with a minimum of five half hitches. Fifteen out of 21 dextrals tied LH or S hitches, the reverse of what Dale Nute found. An ambidextral individual tied mainly S hitches. The two remaining subjects were sinistral. One tied S hitches while the other tied Z hitches. These results suggested that right-handers might favour S hitches, but the disagreement with Nute's findings demonstrated that a much more rigorous investigation was needed.

An additional question was raised by this study. Three of the subjects tied an initial hitch that was the reverse twist or chirality of subsequent hitches. It was not known whether these people could tie the Reef Knot. If they could, was that skill being manifested in these formations? It was also conjectured that, for certain people, the action of tying the initial hitch in a series may be somewhat different from the tying of additional hitches, owing to the number of working ends available or some mechanism their tying habits.

More extensive research has been undertaken in recent decades. Spörri (2008) conducted a detailed survey involving 20 subjects – ten dextrals and ten sinsitrals, as determined by the Edinburgh Handedness Inventory. Right-handed subjects tended to tie predominantly S knots, while left-handed respondents produced mainly S knots, but less frequently than dextrals. She discussed the influence of internal factors – natural tendencies and prior learning – and external factors – such as knot initiation and hand position. Her results agree with previous and later investigations, other than Nute's results as mentioned previously. Spörri also found, through questionnaires, that the incidence of tying sophistication – that is, the use of knots other than simple Overhand Knots and Half Hitches – was very low, and this concurs with other research. Most people in the general population do not tie sophisticated knots that require specialized training or experience.

A qualitative study of the knot tying habits of more than 7,000 people over a period of 25 (Chisnall 2010a) years yielded several key observations that have been guiding subsequent research and forensic investigations of crime-scene evidence. It was noted that tiers tend to have consistent tying habits that are difficult to change, which is in agreement with Nute (Budworth, 1985). Specifically, tiers favoured one enantiomer over the other – tying mainly or exclusively S knots instead of Z knots, for example. Most subjects did not produce sophisticated knot structures, and many who reported being able to tie the Reef or Square Knot did not tie it in practice or could not tie it without difficulty. It was also observed that certain circumstances could cause tiers to switch the chirality of their knots, thus overriding their habit. Switching wends, self-tying, tying overhead, awkward tying situations and obstacles – like long, bulk wends – were observed to produced this chirality-reversal effect.

The most extensive survey of knot-tying habits conducted thus far involved 562 volunteer respondents and thousands of knot samples (Chisnall, 2010b). If every knot tied during the survey is included, regardless of any special conditions, 66% of the knots and hitches tied by dextrals were S, and 56% of those produced by sinistral tiers were Z. In general, left-handers produced Z knots more frequently than right-handers, but not as frequently as dextral tying was dominated by S knots. This agrees with handedness research that found dextrals to be more consistent than sinistrals in uni-manual preference and skill (Crovitz and Zener, 1962; Bryden, 1977; Calvert, 1998).

Since the survey administered required respondents to perform several tying tasks with either one or two wends, it was discovered that switching from two-wend tying to one-wend tying affected the chirality of some tiers' knots. In particular, one-wend tying tasks increased the frequency of S enantiomers up to 75% for dextrals, and the incidence of Z enantiomers up to 63% for sinistrals. Like previous investigations, this study also demonstrated that those claiming to know and use Reef Knots do not always do so. Slightly more than one out of every two respondents claiming Reef skill actually tied one or more Reef Knots. Furthermore, about one in six respondents who indicated they knew how to tie the Reef Knot could actually tie it. Therefore, the fact that an individual produces Reef Knots is not a reliable indicator of tying experience and sophistication. It can be tied innately.

Survey participants were asked to perform a set of two-wend tying tasks: everyday shoelace and parcel tying, the later of which is similar to the creation of crime-scene ligatures. The resulting knots are typically very similar. Either task usually generates pairs of Half Knots in one of four combinations, but shoelace knots incorporate one or two bows or slip loops. Taking into account the tying order of the two Half Knots contained in each task knot, the correlation of knot chirality was moderate. Many residents produced identical parcel and shoelace knots, whether they were S/S or Z/Z Grannies, or S/Z or Z/S Reefs (Figures 6 and 7). However, a significant number deviated from their usual two-wend habit when tying shoelace bows. In fact a small number of tiers completely reversed the chirality of both Half Knots when switching from the parcel-tying task to the shoelace task. Therefore, shoelace knots are not a reliable indication of parcel-tying habits. Task specificity and the number of wends can affect what tiers produce, and prior knowledge and experience may affect their habits. In addition, an intriguing system of sixteen ranked cohorts was revealed, wherein the pattern for sinistrals was nearly the mirror image of that for dextrals, as determined by the Spearman rank correlation coefficient and the Signed Rank Test (Chisnall, 2010a).

Additional data acquired from the same survey (Chisnall, 2009) indicated that 3% of the tiers surveyed produce unusual anomalies – like Figure Eight and Figure Nine Hitches, which are not illustrated – particularly when tying bows or slip loops. This lends credence to the notion that special or unusual tying tasks or situations may influence a tier's basic knot-tying tendencies.

An analysis of 114 cases and 584 distinct knots confirmed many of these observations (Chisnall, 2011). Where it could be verified, single tiers were consistent in their tying habits and the chirality of their knots, which corroborates Nute's observations (Budworth, 1985). Additionally, most of the tiers of those case knots did not have any sophisticated knot-tying skill (Chisnall, 2011), further confirming previous observations (Chisnall, 2010a; 2010b).

All of the information derived from surveys and other research could be useful in certain forensic investigations, but a very fundamental and important notion has emerged. Whereas classical knot-craft is an esoteric study of knot forms, functions, and lore, forensic knot investigation is related to behavioural science. The knots used in crimes are comparatively basic and unremarkable. However, the actions of the tier, his or her motivations and knowledge, and the tying situations that occur during criminal activity can be complex. The knots preserved are valuable exhibits that serve as a record of that tier's behaviour.

Forensic Science Applications

Insights derived from surveys, case work and other research assist forensic investigators and litigators in a number of ways (Polson and Gee, 1967; Simpson, 1985; Budworth, 1982a; 1982b; Nute, 1986; Hazelwood, et al., 1981; Chisnall, 2000; 2007). Exhibits acquired from death and crime scenes, at the most basic practical level, provide grounds for search warrants and wire tapes when hunting for suspects and other evidence. The arrangements of knots and ligatures may offer clues that will assist crime-scene analysts in reconstructing the crime-scene events as well as distinguishing between suicide, homicide, auto-erotic fatalities, homicide disguised as suicide and so forth.

At a deeper level, the knots and ligatures may indicate whether one or more tiers were involved and afford clues as to the characteristics of the tiers, such as handedness and knotting experience and skill. However, as the research data clearly demonstrate, the link between basic knot enantiomers and tier handedness is not binary and is often equivocal. Knot evidence cannot be used with the same statistical certainty as finger print or DNA evidence. There is no such thing as a signature knot. Knot exhibits must be regarded as group-or class-characteristic evidence and, therefore, such evidence best suited to corroborate other facts and evidence germane to any case in question (Tuthill, 1994; Chisnall, 2000).

It is hoped that the current trend research into knot-tying habits will increase investigator confidence in the proper analysis of knotted evidence, extend or solidify the scope and range of the field, and evolve to satisfy the emerging requirements for statistical rigour, especially regarding the use of Bayesian statistics when assessing crime-scene exhibits and suspect knot samples.

Linking Knot-Tying Habits to Handedness: Speculations and Further Research

The research pertaining to knot-tying behaviour that has accumulated to date offers several useful revelations, all of which serve to inform and guide the conscientious investigator of knotted evidence. Here is a summary of what has been repeatedly observed:

- S enantiomers occurred more frequently than their Z counterparts in surveys of everyday tying tasks and in case evidence.
- Individuals identified as right-handers tied S more frequently than Z enantiomers. However, the correlation is more complex than a simple binary relationship.
- Other factors – like the number of wends utilized in the tying task – influenced the chirality of the knots produced. For example, some tiers will prefer S knots when using two wends, but they will switch to Z when using one wend.
- Individuals identified as left-handers tended to tie Z more frequently in certain tasks and S more frequently in others. However, the frequency of

S enantiomers in sinistral tying was lower than the frequency of S enantiomers exhibited in dextral tying. (This may be related to the fact that dextrals are more strongly right-handed in their uni-manual skills than sinsitrals are left-handed in their skill preferences.)

- Extenuating factors, such as the tying of bows or slips loops, awkward tying positions, unusual rope or cord characteristics, and interference may influence a tier's habits by causing reversals in enantiomer chirality. Self-tying and overhead tying can have a similar effect.

Most important, as it related to handedness research, the research data suggest that there is a gradation of knot-tying behaviours that may be correlated with the spectrum of hand dominance across the general population. Future inquiries may show that those who exhibit strong or exclusive dextral dominance prefer S in most tying tasks, while those who are primarily left-handed will prefer Z knots most of the time. Between those two extremes, a shared preference for S and Z in specific tasks may be correlated with degrees of hand dominance (inconsistent, mixed or shared handedness).

It might be appropriate to incorporate standardized knot-tying tasks into the battery of manual tests researchers administer to analyse hand preference because basic knot tying is sensitive to the direction of the twisting or wrapping movements the dominant hand performs. Informative patterns may be observed if attention is paid to the chirality of the knots themselves, which, as illustrated previously, has been ignored in previous work (Tracy, 2003; Leff, et al., 2006; 2008).

Although Burt and Blau's early work pertaining to the psychopathology of left-handedness was flawed and has been criticised (Harris, 1980; Boake, et al., 1983; Beaton, 1985; Charlton, 1988), it might offer something of value. The classic Blau torque test, which examines whether respondents make circles in a clockwise or anticlockwise direction with either hand, could be linked to knot-tying actions. The uni-manual movements associated with wrapping a cord or rope wend in an S or Z fashion could be related or similar to clockwise and counterclockwise wrist and lower arm writing motions. Although not a precise determinant of brain laterality, this Blau torque test suggests that if a respondent draws counterclockwise circles with both hands, they likely possess left-hemispheric dominance and are therefore dextral. If an individual produces clockwise circles, they have right hemispheric dominance and are left-handed. If a respondent produces some combination of clockwise and counterclockwise circles, that person likely has shared dominance, or so the test is purported to indicate. The question is, how relevant and useful might this connection be to investigations of knot-tying habits and modern research in neuropsychology?

In the early stages of the extensive knot-tying survey previously described (Chisnall, 2009; 2010b), some comparative data was collected that has been hitherto unreported. Out of the more than 500 respondents who volunteered for the study, an initial 105 were asked to undertake the Blau torque test in conjunction with the various knot tasks in that survey. The data are summarized in Table 1 and, although inconclusive, beg further investigation. There were not enough sinistral and ambidextral survey participants to generate any discernible patterns, but those respondents deemed primarily right-handed were more abundant in the CC/CC cohort and they tended to prefer S enantiomers, as mentioned earlier. A more extensive study, involving a much higher number of participants, could shed light on the relationship between handedness, tying habits and circling behaviour. It would be informative to utilize a multivariate analysis technique and compare these three variables across three axes of gradation.

Table 1. A comparison of participant handedness (using criteria similar to Annett's 1970 Handedness Inventory), knot-tying habits (tying multiple S or Z enantiomers over several tasks), and the Blau torque test results (drawing three circles with each hand). The data indicate the numbers of respondents in each cohort out of a total of 105 survey participants

Blau Torque Test Outcome	CC/CC		CC/C		C/CC		C/C	
Principal Enantiomer Chirality	S	Z	S	Z	S	Z	S	Z
Number of Mainly Right Handed-Respondents	39	16	23	8	4	2	2	3
Number of Ambidextral Respondents	1	1	2*					
Number of Mainly Left-Handed Respondents	1	1		1			1	

S = Tied all or mostly S Overhand Knots, Half Hitches or Half Knots.
Z = Tied all or mostly Z Overhand Knots, Half Hitches or Half Knots.
CC/CC = Circled three times with both hands in a counterclockwise direction.
CC/C = Circled counterclockwise with the left hand and clockwise with the right hand.
C/CC = Circled clockwise with the left hand and counterclockwise with the right hand.
C/C = Circled three time with both hands in a clockwise direction.
* Both respondents tied S and Z knots equally.

Similar to the many physiological, genetic, sociological and experiential factors that impinge on each individual's handedness, knot-tying habits may be a product of several interacting external and internal phenomena. Adapted from Spörri (2008), Figure 15 charts a behavioural model detailing the process of tying a knot. This model specifically applies to crime-scene knot investigations, but the same factors listed come into play during commonplace tying and they should be considered when knot-tying tasks are part of any behavioural study.

Expanded Model:

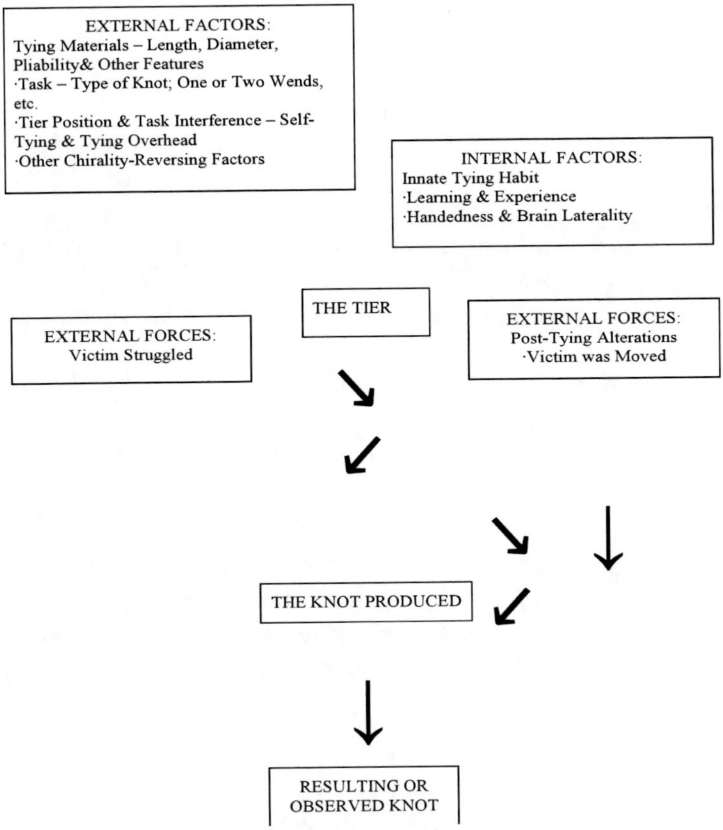

Spörri's Original Model:
External and Internal Factors → Tier → Resulting Knot → External Forces → Observed Knot.

Figure 15. A conceptual model for understanding and analysing tying behaviour in terms of initial factors and outcomes. This flow chart is adapted from a simpler version presented by Spörri (2008, p. 29). Extra detail has been provided at those stages research has shown to be influential.

Conclusion

To date, handedness research has informed and directed initial investigations into tying habits. Future research inquiries may well benefit from examining trends and action specificity in basic tying tasks to uncover more details regarding the underlying mechanisms of handedness and the learning of asymmetrical or uni-manual skills.

There are at least two lessons that can be drawn from this discussion. First, is it clear that prior research in neuropsychology and related fields ignored knot chirality when incorporating tying tasks into the research protocol. Evidence suggests that chirality could have a significant influence on the tier's behaviour, since tiers tend to favour either S or Z enantiomers. In particular, if a test subject is being taught to tie a specific knot as part of the experimental procedure, the investigator should be sensitive to that person's innate tying habits and how forcing contrary forms through training may influence their behaviour and cloud the research issue in question.

Second, the case can be made that simple tying tasks could be feasibly combined with handedness-defining tasks and incorporated into various laterality-determining questionnaires and inventories. Of course consideration but be paid to the exact nature of the knot-tying tasks utilized – whether tying with one or two wends, and so forth. However revealing this might be, it will add complexity to investigations. Clearly, more work is required before the knot-tying profile of research subjects can be used in an informative way. At present, our understanding of handedness and tying habits is self-referential and circular. Whatever handedness suggests about tying habits, and vice versa, is a two-way street with several complicating factors yet to be unravelled in conjunction with the larger realm of handedness research. What emerges should benefit both the fields of psychology and forensic science.

References

Annett, M. (1967). The binomial distribution of right, mixed and left handers. *Quarterly Journal of Experimental Psychology, 19*, 327-334.

Annett, M. (1970). A classification of hand preference by association analysis. *British Journal of Psychology,* 61 (3), 303-321.

Annett, M. (1972). The distribution of manual asymmetry. *British Journal of Psychology,* 63, 343-358.

Annett, M. (1973). Handedness in families. *Annals of Human Genetics,* 37 (1), 93-105.

Annett, M. (1974). Handedness in the children of two left-handed parents. *British Journal of Psychology,* 65, 129-131.

Annett, M. (1978). Genetic and nongenetic influences on handedness. *Behavior Genetics,* 8 (3), 227-249.

Annett, J., Annett, M., Hudson, P.T.W., and Turner, A. (1979). The control of movements in the preferred and non-preferred hands. *Quarterly Journal of Experimental Psychology,* 31, 641-652.

Annett M. (1992). Five tests of hand skill. *Cortex,* 28, 583-600.

Ashley, C. W. (1944). *The Ashlev Book of Knots.* Garden City, New York: Doubleday and Company, Inc.

Baldwin, J. (1890). Origin of right or left handedness. *Science,* 16, 2, 47-248.

Baldwin, J. (1894). The origin of right-handedness. *Popular Science Monthly,* 44, 606-615.

Balter, Michael. (2009). The origins of handedness, *The Science of Origins. American Association for the Advancement of Science.* Posted August 18, 2009 at http://sciencemag.org/origins/2009/08/the-origins-of-handedness.html

Barsley, M. (1966). *The Other Hand: An Investigation Into the Sinister History of Left-handedness.* New York: Hawthorn.

Barsley, M. (1970). *Left-handed Man in a Right-handed World.* London, Great Britain: Pitman Publishing.

Beaton, A. (1985). *Left Side, Right Side.* New Haven, Connecticut: Yale University Press.

Beck, L.F. (1936). Manual skills and the measurement of handedness. *The Journal of Psychology,* 2, 259-272.

Beeley, A. L. (1919). Left-handedness. *American Journal of Physical Anthropology,* 2, 389-400.

Boake, C., Salmon, P. G., and Carbone, G. (1983). Torque, lateral preference, and cognitive ability in primary-grade children. *Journal of Abnormal Child Psychology,* 11 (1), 77-83

Bonaparte, M., Freud, A., Kris, E. (Eds.) (1954). *The Origins of Psychoanalysis: Letters to Wilhelm Fliess, Drafts, and Notes, 1887-1902 by Sigmund Freud.* New York: Basic Books.

Briggs, G. G., Nebes, R. D. Patterns of hand preference in a student populations. *Cortex,* 11 (3),230-8.

Brewster, E. T. (1913). *The ways of the left hand.* McClure's Magazine, 41 (June), 168-183.

Briggs, G.G., Nebes, R.D. (1975). Patterns of hand preference in a student population, *Cortex,* 11(3): 230-238.

Brown, S., Roy, E., Rohr, L., and Bryden, P. (2006). Using hand performance measures to predict handedness. *Laterality: Asymmetries of Body, Brain, and Cognition*, 11 (1), 1-14.

Bryden, M. P. (1977). *Measuring handedness with questionnaires. Neuropsychologia,* 15, 617-624.

Budworth, G. (1982a). Identification of Knots. *Journal of the Forensic Science Society,* 22, 327-331.

Budworth, G. (1982b). *The Identification of Knots.* London, England: Metropolitan Police Force Forensic Science Laboratory.

Budworth, G. (1985). *Knots and Crime.* Letchworth, Great Britain: Police Review Publishing Co. Ltd.

Buchanan, A. (1862). Mechanical theory of the preponderance of the right hand of the left; or, more generally, of the limbs of the right side over the left side of the body. *Proceedings* of the . Philosophical Society of Glasgow, 5, 142-107.

Burt, C. (1937). *The Backward Child.* London, England: University of London Press.

Calvert G. A. (1998). Quantifying hand preference using a behavioural continuum. *Laterality: Asymmetries of Body, Brain and Cognition,* 3 (3), 255-268.

Canadian Government Specifications Board. (1978). *Standards 40-GP-1M.* [Place of publication unknown.]

Canadian General Standards Board. (1984). *Standards CAN2-4.2-M77*, Method 9.4. [Place of publication unknown.]

Caron-Pargue, J. (1983). Codage verbal et codage graphique de noeuds. [Verbal coding and graphical coding of knots.] *In Groupe de Reserche Ontogénèse des Processus Psychologiques,* La Pensée Naturelle: Structures, Procédures et Logique du Sujet (pp. 44-52.) Paris: Publications de L'Université de Rouen.

Caron-Pargue, J. (1985). Analyse d'instructions graphiques pour faire un noeud: La filiation des significations dans des dessins d'enfants. [*Analysis of knot-tying instructions: the correspondence of intended meaning in children's drawings.*] Unpublished paper, Laboratoire de Psychologie, Université de Rouen.

Carter-Saltzman, L. (1980). Biological and sociocultural effects on handedness: comparison between biological and adoptive families. *Science,* 209 (4462), 1263-1265.

Casey, M. B., Brabeck, M.M., and Ludlow, L. H. (1986). Familial handedness and its relation to spatial ability following strategy instructions. *Intelligence,* 10, 389-406.

Chamberlain, H. D. (1928). The inheritance of left-handedness. *Journal of Heredity,* 19, 557-559.

Charlton, S. (1988). Torque and cerebral laterlization: a questionable link. *International Journal of Neuroscience,* 43 (1-2), 15-19.

Chisnall, R. (1994). A survey of tier handedness and habit – some preliminary data. *Knotting Matters,* 45, 9-14.

Chisnall R. (2000). *The Forensic Analysis of Knots and Ligatures.* Salem, Oregon: Lightning Powder Company, Inc.

Chisnall R. (2007). What knots can reveal: the strengths and limitations of forensic knot analysis. *Journal of Forensic Identification,* 57 (5), 726-749.

Chisnall R. (2009). Tying anomalies and their significance in analysing knot evidence. *Canadian Society of Forensic Science Journal,* 42 (3), 172-194.

Chisnall R. (2010a). Knot-tying habits, tier handedness and experience. *J Forensic Sci.* 2010;55(5):1232-1244.

Chisnall R. (2010b). Basic Principles of Forensic Knot Analysis: A Qualitative Study of Tying Behaviour. *Investigative Sciences Journal,* 2 (3), 33-44.

Chisnall, R. (2011.) An analysis of more than 100 cases involving knots and ligatures: knot frequencies, consistent tying habits and noteworthy outliers. *Australian Journal of Forensic Sciences.* In press.

Clark, M.M. (1974). *Teaching Left-Handed Children.* London, England: University of London Press Ltd.

Collins, R. L. (1988). Observational learning of a left right asymmetry by mice (Mus musculus). *Journal of Comparative Psychology,* 102, 222-224.

Corballis, M.C. (1980). Is left-handedness genetically determined? In *J. Herron* (Ed.), *Neuropsychology of Left-handedness* (pp. 159-176). New York: Academic Press.

Coren, S. and Porac, C. (1979). Normative data on hand position during writing. *Coretex,* 15, 679-682.

Corey D. M., Hurley M.M., and Foundas A. L. (2001). Right and left handedness defined: a multivariate approach using hand preference and hand performance measures. Neuropsychiatry, *Neuropsychology and Behavioral Neurology,* 14 (3),144-52.

Crichton-Browne, J. (1907). Dexterity and the bend sinister. *Proceedings of the Royal Institution of Great Britain,* 18, 623-652.

Crovitz, H. and Zener, K. (1962). A group test for assessing hand-and-eye dominance. *American Journal of Psychology,* 75, 271-276.

Dragovic M, Hammond G. A classification of handedness using the Annett hand preference questionnaire. *British Journal of Psychology,* 98 (3), 375-87.

Doyen, A. L., and Carlier. M. (2001). Measuring handedness: a validation study of Bishop's reaching card test. *Laterality: Asymmetries of Body, Brain, and Cognition,* 7 (2), 115-130.

Doyen, A. L., Duquenne, V., Nuques, S., and Carlier, M. (2004). What can be learned from a lattice analysis of a laterality questionnaire? *Behavior Genetics,* 31 (2), 193-207.

Eliot, J., and Salking, N. J., (Eds.) (1975). *Children's Spatial Development.* Springfield, Illinois: Charles C. Thomas.

Flowers, K. (1975). Handedness and controlled movement. *British Journal of Psychology,* 66 (1), 39-52.

Flowers, K. (1983). Manual performance asymmetries and motor control processes: subject-generated changes in response parameters. *Human Movement Science,* 2 (4)271-277.

Francks, C., Margawa, S., Laurén, J., Abrahams, B.S., Velayos-Baeza, A., Meland, S.E., Colella, S., Groszer, M., MaAuley, E.Z., et al. (2007). LRRTM1 on chromosome 2p12 is a maternally suppressed gene that is associated paternally with handedness and schizophrenia.. *Journal of Molecular Psychiatry,* 12 (12), 1129-1139.

Hannaford, C. (2005). *Smart Moves: Why Learning is Not All in Your Head.* Salt Lake City: Great River Books.

Harris, L. J. (1980). Left-handedness: early theories, facts, and fancies. In Herron, J. (Ed.), *Neuropsychology of Left-handedness* (pp. 3-78). New York: Academic Press.

Hartlage, L. C., and Gage, R. (1997). Unimanual performance as a measure of laterality. *Neuropsychology Review*, 7 (3), 143-156.

Hazelwood, R., Dietz, A. E., and Berges, A. W. (1981). *Autoerotic Fatalities.* Toronto, Canada: Lexicon Books.

Hepper, P. G., McCartney, G.R., and Shannon, E.A. (1998). Lateralized behaviour in first trimester human fetuses. *Neuropsychologia* 36, 531-534.

Herron, Jeannine (Ed.). (1980). *Neuropsychology of Left-handedness.* New York: Academic Press.

Herzfeld, C, and Lestel, D. (2006). Knot tying in great apes: etho-ethnology of an unusual tool behavior. *Social Science Information,* 44 (4) 621-653.

Hopkins, W. D., Dunham, L., Cantalupo, C., and Taglialatela, J. (2007). The association between handedness, brain asymmetry and corpus callosum size in chimpanzees (Pan troglodytes). *Cerebral Cortex,* 17 (8), 1757-1765.

Hopkins, W. D., and Russell, J. L. (2004). Further evidence of a right hand advantage in motor skills by chimpanzees (Pan troglodytes), *Neuropsychologia,* 42 (7), 2004, 990-996.

Ide R. (2009). Knots under the microscope. *Knotting Matters,* 103, 24-27.

Jackson, J. (1905). *Ambidexterity or Two-handedness and Two-brainedness.* London, England: Kegan Paul, Trench, Trubner and Co., Ltd.

Jordan, H. E. (1911). The inheritance of left-handedness. *American Breeder's Magazine,* 2, 19-28; 113-124.

Jordan, H. E. (1922). The crime against left-handedness. *Good Health,* 57, 378-383.

Jordan, T. R., Patching, G. R. (2003). Assessing the role of hemispheric specialisation, serial-position processing, and retinal eccentricity in lateralised word recognition, *Cognitive Neuropsychology*, 2003, 20 (1), 49-71.

Kimura, D. and Vanderwolf, C.H. (1970). The relation between hand preference and the performance of individual finger movements by left and right hands. *Brain,* 93, 769-774.

Laska, M. (1996). Manual laterality in spider monkeys (Ateles geoffroyi) solving visual and tactually guided food-reaching tasks. *Cortex* 32 (4), 717-726.

Leff, D., Koh, P. H., Aggarwal, R., Leong, J., Deligiani, F., Elwell, C., Delpy, D. T., Darzi, A., and Yang, G. Z. (2006). Optical mapping of the frontal cortex during a surgical knot-tying task, a feasibility study. *Lecture Notes in Computer Science,* 4091, 140-148.

Leff, D., Elwell, R.C., Orihuela-Espina, F., Atallah, L., Delpy, D. T., Darzi, A. W., and Yang, G. Z.. (2008). Changes in prefrontal cortical behaviour depend upon familiarity on a bimanual co-ordination task: an fNIS study. *NeoImage,* 39 (2), 805-813.

Levy, J. and Nagylaki, T. (1972). *A model for genetics of the hand. Genetics*, 72, 117-128.

Levy, J. and Reid, M. L. (1976) Variations in writing posture and cerebral organization. *Science,* 194, 337-339.

Loo, R., and Schneider, R. (1979). An evaluation of the Briggs-Nebes modified version of Annett's handedness inventory. *Cortex,* 15 (4), 683-686.

McCartney, G. R., and Hepper, P.G. (1999). Development of laterized behaviour in the human fetus from 12-27 weeks' gestation. *Developmental Medicine and Child Neurology,* 41, 83-86

Miller, E. (1971). Handedness and the pattern of human ability. *British Journal of Psychology,* 7, 19-48.

Michel, George F., Harkins, Debra A. (1985). Concordance of handedness between teachers and student facilitates Learning Manual skills. *Journal of Human Evolution,* 14, (6), 597-601.

Moscovitch. M., and Smith, L.C. (1979). Differences in neural organisation between individuals with inverted and non-inverted handwriting postures. *Science,* 205, 710-712.

Nakamura, R., and Saito, H. (1974). Preferred hand and reaction time in different movement patterns. *Perceptual and Motor Skills,* 39, 1275-1281.

Netley, C. (1988). Relationships between hemispheric lateralization, sex hormones, quality of parenting and adjustment in 47, XXY males prior to puberty. *Journal of Child Psychology and Psychiatry,* 29 (3), 282-287.

Nice, M.M. (1918). Ambidexterity and delayed speech development. *Pedagogical Seminary,* 25, 141-162.

Nute, H. D. (1986). Mirror images in knots. *Journal of Forensic Sciences,* 31 (1), 272-279.

Oldfield, R. C. (1971) The assessment of handedness: the Edinburgh inventory. *Neuropsychologia,* 9, 97-113.

Olson, D. R. (1970). *Cognitive Development: The Child's Acquisition of Diagonality*. New York: Academic Press.

Overstreet, R. (1938). An investigation of prenatal position and handedness. *Psychological Bulletin,* 35, 520-521.

Parlow, S. (1978). Differential finger movements and hand preference. *Cortex,* 14, 608-611.

Pawson, D. (1992). Left hand - right hand? *Knotting Matters.* 41, 14.

Peters, M. (1981). Handedness effect of prolonged practice on between hand performance differences. *Neuropsychologia,* 19, 570-590.

Peters, M. and Durding, B. M. (1978). Handedness measured by finger tapping: a continuous variable. *Canadian Journal of Psychology,* 32, 257-261.

Piaget, J. (1951). *The Child's Conception of the World.* Translated by J. and A. Tomlinson, J. and Tomlinson, A. (Translators), New York: Humanities Press. (Originally published in 1929).

Piaget, J., and Inhelder, B.. (1967). *The Child's Conception of Space.* Langdon, F.J., and Lunzer, J.L. (Translators). New York: W.W. Norton. (Originally published in 1948).

Piaget, J. (1977). *The Essential Piaget.* Gruber, H. E., and Vonèche, J.J. (Eds.). New York: Basic Books.

Polson, C. J., and Gee, D. J. (1973). *The Essentials of Forensic Medicine,* Third Edition. Toronto: Pergamon Press.

Provins, K. A. (1967). Motor skills, handedness and behaviour. *Australian Journal of Psychology,* 19, 137-150.

Ramaley, F. (1913). Inheritance of left-handedness. *American Naturalist*, 47, 730-738.

Ramsay, D. S. (1980). Onset of unimanual handedness in infants. *Infant Behaviour and Development,* 3, 377-385.

Ransil, B. J., Schachter, S.C. (1994). Test-re test reliability of the Edinburgh Handedness Inventory and global handedness preference measurements, and their correlation. *Perceptual and Motor Skills,* 79 (1), 1355-1372.

Rife, D. C. (1940). Handedness, with special reference to twins. *Genetics,* 25, 178-186.

Sainburg, R. L. (2002). Evidence for dynamic-dominance hypothesis of handedness. *Experimental Brain Research,* 142, 241-258, 2002.

Sainburg, R. L., and Schaefer, S. Y. (2004). Interlimb differences in control of movement extent. *Journal of Neurophysiology,* 92, 1374-1383.

Satz, P. (1972). Pathological left-handedness: An explanatory model. *Cortex,* 8, 121-135.

Shanon, B. (1978). Writing positions in Americans and Israelis. *Neuropsychologia,* 16, 587-591.

Schulter-Ellis, F.P. (1980). Evidence of handedness on documented skeletons. *Journal of Forensic Sciences,* 25 (3), 624-630.

Siebner, H. R., Limmer, C., Peinemann, A., Drzezga, A., Bloem, B. R., Schwaiger, M., and Conrad, B. (2002). Long-term consequences of switching handedness: a positron emission tomography study on handwriting in "converted" left-handers. *The Journal of Neuroscience,* 22 (7), 2816-2825.

Silverstein, A. and Silverstein, V.B. (1977). *The Left-Hander's World.* Chicago: Follet Publishing.

Simpson, K. (1985). *Forensic Medicine,* Ninth Edition. London, England: Edward Arnold (Publishers) Ltd.

Smith, L. G. (1917). A brief survey of right- and left-handedness. *Pedagogical Seminary,* 24, 19-35.

Spörri S. (2008). La valeur indiciale des noeuds. [The indicative value of knots]. *Unpublished dissertation.* Lausanne-Dorigny, Switzerland: University of Lausanne, Ecole des sciences criminelles, Institut de Police Scientifique.

Steenhuis, R. E., and Bryden, M. P. (1989). Different dimensions of hand preference that relate to skilled and unskilled activities. *Cortex,* 25 (2), 289-304.

Steingruber, H.J. (1975). Handedness as a function of test complexity. *Perceptual and Motor Skills,* 40, 263-266.

Steinmetz, H., Volkmann, J., Jäncke, L., and Freund, H.J. (1991). Anatomical left-right asymmetry of language-related temporal cortex is different in left- and right-handers, *Anals of Neurology,* 29 (3), 315-319.

Strohecker, C. (1996). Understanding topological relationships through comparisons of similar knots. *AI and Society,* 10 (1), 58-69.

Strohecker, C. (1991). *Why Knot?* Unpublished doctoral dissertation. Cambridge, Massachusetts:

Massachusetts Institute of Technology, *Media Laboratory.*

Strohecker, C. (1990). *Knot-Tying: A Constructionist Environment for Topology.* Unpublished paper. Cambridge, Massachusetts: Massachusetts Institute of Technology, Media Laboratory.

Strohecker, C. (1989a). *The Knot Lab: Protocol on Construction of the Family Tree.* Unpublished paper. Cambridge, Massachusetts: Massachusetts Institute of Technology, Media Laboratory.

Strohecker, C. (1989)b. *The Knot Lab: PT's Case Study. Unpublished paper.* Cambridge, Massachusetts: Massachusetts Institute of Technology, Media Laboratory.

Strohecker, C. (1989c). *The Knot Lab: Case Studies. Unpublished paper.* Cambridge, Massachusetts: Massachusetts Institute of Technology, Media Laboratory. Massachusetts Institute of Technology.

Sumners, D. W. (1987). *The role of knot theory in DNA research.* In McCory, C. and Shifrin, T. (Eds.), Geometry and Topology: Manifolds, Varieties and Knots. Lecture Notes in Pure and Applied Mathematics, 105, 297-318, New York: Dekker.

Sun, T., and Alsh, C. A. (2006). Molecular level brain asymmetry. *Nature Reviews Neurosceince,* 7, 655-662.

Tichy, J., and Belacek, J. (2009). Laterality in children: cerebellar dominance, handedness, footedness and hair whorl. *Activitas Nervosa Superior Rediviva,* 51, (1-2), 9-20.

Todor, J. I., and Doane, T. (1977). Handedness classification: preference versus proficiency. *Perceptual and Motor Skills,* 45, 1041-1041.

Tracy, J., Flanders, A., Madi, S., Laskas, J., Stoddard E., Pyrros, A., Natale, P., and DelVecchio, N. (2003). Regional brain activation associated with different performance patterns during learning of a complex motor skill. *Cerebral Cortex,* 13 (9), 904-910.

Trankell, A. (1955). Aspects of genetics in psychology. *American Journal of Human Genetics,* 7, 264-276.

Tuthill, H. (1994). *Individualization: Principles and Procedures in Criminalistics.* Salem, Oregon: Lightning Powder Company, Inc.

Underwood, R. (1988). *Personal correspondence.*

Uomini, N. T. (2009). The prehistory of handedness: archeological data and comparative ethology. *Journal of Human Evolution,* 57 (4), 411-419.

van der Kleij, G. (1996). Chapter 3. On Knots and Swamps: Knots in European Prehistory. In Turner, J.C., and van de Griend, P. (Eds.), *History and Science of Knots: Series on Knots and Everything,* (Volume 11, pp. 43-68). New Jersey: World Scientific.

Verdino M, Dingman, S. (1998). Two measures of laterality in handedness: the Edinburgh Handedness Inventory and the Purdue Pegboard Test of manual dexterity. *Perceptual and Motor Skills,* 86 (20), 476-8.

Warner, C. (1996). Why Knot? - Some Speculations on the Earliest Knots. In Turner, J.C., and van de Griend, P. (Eds.), History and Science of Knots: Series on Knots and Everything, (Volume 11, pp. 43-68). New Jersey: *World Scientific.*

Warner, C. , and Bednarik, R. G. (1996). Chapter 1. Pleistocene Knotting. In Turner, J.C., and van de Griend, P. (Eds.), *History and Science of Knots: Series on Knots and Everything,* (Volume 11, pp. 43-68). New Jersey: World Scientific.

Wendrich, W. (1996). Chapter 4. Ancient Egyptian Rope and Knots. In Turner, J. C., and van de Griend, P. (Eds.), *History and Science of Knots: Series on Knots and Everything,* (Volume 11, pp. 43-68). New Jersey: World Scientific.

Wilson, P. T., and Jones, H. E. (1932). *Left-handedness in twins. Genetics,* 17, 560-571.

Witelson, S. F., and Pallie, W. (1973). Left hemisphere specialization for language in the newborn: neuroanatomical evidence of asymmetry. *Brain,* 96, 641-646.

Woolley, H. T. (1910). The development of right-handedness in a normal infant. *Psychological Review,* 17, 37-41.

In: Handedness: Theories, Genetics and Psychology ISBN: 978-1-61470-502-4
Editors: J. Dunham and T. Davenport

Chapter II

A Brief History of Handedness Research

Robert Chisnall
Faculty of Education, Queen's University, Kingston, Ontario, Canada

Abstract

Manual asymmetry has long fascinated investigators, and the rarity of left-handed individuals in the general population has been a puzzle. Researchers have endeavoured to answer three fundamental questions:

- What is handedness?
- How can it be measured?
- What are its mechanisms?

These questions delve into the very nature of brain function and they have served to guide psychologists, educators, physicians, therapists, physiologists and other scientists in their quest to unravel numerous mysteries. What follows is a brief historical outline of theories that gave rise to current behavioural, genetic, and physiological models of laterality and handedness.

Anthropological and Historical Overview

Initial theories of handedness were sensitive to the statistical rarity of sinistrality. Modern theories are no different in that respect. However, early researchers concerned themselves with any historical or anthropological evidence that could be gleaned from a variety of sources. It was thought that if consistent commonness of right-handedness could be determined, and roughly the same proportions occurred throughout all cultures and historical periods, then the underlying factor was biological. Conversely, if the proportion of dextrals and sinistrals could be shown to vary with social and technical changes, then handedness could be attributed to cultural influences. The classic nature-nurture controversy fuelled the philosophy and methodology of early research. Analysing artefacts from prehistoric societies, and observing primate behaviour were and still are two useful approaches to this research problem (Laska, 1996; Warner and Bednarik, 1996; Hopkins and Russell, 2004; Hopkins, et al., 2007; Herzfeld and Lestel, 2006).

The literature variously reports that dextrality constitutes anywhere from 65% to 95% of the general human population (Michel and Harkins, 1985; Hannaford, 2005). Although, as Uomini (2009) reported, 85% of Homo sapiens are right-handed for most uni-manual actions, other great ape species do not display consistent laterlization. Evidence suggests that human dextrality may have emerged at the species level through the social transmission of increasingly complex tool use activities, wherein there is bimanual differentiation. There is clear evidence (Balter, 2009) from numerous Neanderthal skeletons that those prehistoric hominids tended to be right-handed. Detailed measurements of the dorsal inclination of the glenoid fossa, humeral length and head diameter, length and width, and radial and ulnar lengths can be used to determine handedness (Schulter-Ellis, 1980). Studies of human and nonhuman primates suggest that handedness varies in accordance with the complexity of the task and the skill level required to perform it (William, et al., 2007; Uonomi, 2009; Balter, 2009).

The indirect evidence of other Stone Age artifacts was ambiguous at times. The pattern of chipping on hand axes and tools showed that some were made by left-handers, others by right-handers (Silverstein and Silverstein, 1977). Cave paintings from Europe's Mammoth and Reindeer Periods gave further clues (Harris, 1980). A right-handed individual tends to draw figures and heads facing left when depicted in profile; left-handers find it easier to draw right-facing profiles (Silverstein and Silverstein, 1977). Both types of renderings were found in ancient paintings. Overall, the evidence was inconclusive and confusing. Prehistoric people were either ambidextrous or equally left- and right-handed.

There is agreement that right-handedness has predominated since the Old Testament (Harris, 1980). The Bible itself served as a source of evidence, although interpretations of the notable passages in Genesis, Psalms and Judges generated debate owing to differing translations.

Tools and weapons acquired from the Bronze Age or later indicated the preeminence of the right hand (Silverstein and Silverstein, 1977). The Teta tomb at Gizeh (2,200 B.C.) houses stone carvings that show the right hand in an attitude of supplication. Bas-reliefs of ancient Assyrians and Cambodians highlighted the dominance of the right hand in wielding a sword (Harris, 1980). Many explanations were offered. It was speculated that a sword or spear held in an attacker's right-hand would have a better chance of piercing his enemy's leftward slanting heart, while the shield held in the left hand would better protect that more vulnerable side of the body (Silverstein and Silverstein, 1977). This was regarded as a weak theory because the slight leftward slant of the heart is actually insignificant.

Evidence distilled from the artifacts and ruins of ancient Egyptians, Greeks, and Romans also lent credence to the notion that right-handedness was the norm during historical times (Silverstein and Silverstein, 1977; Wendrich, 1996). However, exact numbers could not be established.

The determination of a constant and universal proportion in population handedness was impossible, and this was frustrating for researchers. To discover ambiguities and inconsistencies in the anthropological and historical evidence was to generate more unanswered questions. A simple choice between cultural and biological mechanisms could not be made (Harris, 1980).

Theories combining physiological and societal explanations did develop though.

Early Theories

Early explanations of handedness can be divided into five main categories (Harris, 1980):

- those stressing structural asymmetries of the human body;
- theories linking handedness to cultural conditioning and learning;
- the search for hereditary mechanisms;

- speculations attributing handedness to a pathological state of brain or personality;
- and attributions of left-handedness to statistical rarity.

By modern standards, some of these approaches seem silly. It has taken years of careful research to dispel the prejudices and fallacies inherent in such notions, ideas that often hindered scientific inquiry or clouded emerging facts. However, some ideas were grounded in sound reasoning and they persist today as bases for more elaborate hypotheses.

Structural Asymmetry

Several prominent scientists of the 1800's suggested handedness could be explained by the asymmetrical arrangement of internal organs like the heart and liver. If these organs appeared as the mirror image of the normal visceral pattern, then the individual in question would be left-handed (Harris, 1980). With only vague clinical support, this theory became the subject of much discussion throughout European medical circles. It was all but forgotten eighty years later. However, visceral asymmetry remained a popular foundation for subsequent ideas.

Andrew Buchanan advanced a theory in 1862 that became well known (Beaton, 1985). He focussed on the asymmetry of the lungs and liver. The great weight of the liver was conjectured to cause a shift in balance to the left side, leaving the limbs on the right-hand side freer for action. Borelli and Weber used cadavers to make determinations regarding centre of balance, but nothing conclusive could be said about whether this point was situated in or displaced from the mesial plane relative to handedness (Harris, 1980; Netley, 1988). Several researchers of the period attempted to link this theory with embryology, but criticisms of visceral asymmetry as a theoretical base were frequent and harsh.

For several centuries, up until the 19th Century, certain blood-flow theories were pushed as explanations for handedness (Beaton, 1985). It was thought that differential blood flow to the arms was the cause of hand dominance. This idea, often called the 'subclavian theory' after the artery, did not survive when it was increasingly recognized in the 18th Century that the hemispheres of the brain and not the hands were the critical organs (Harris, 1980).

The work of Paul Broca (1827-1880) and anatomical characteristics of aphasic patients gave impetus to investigations of brain specialization. It was discovered that the third frontal convolution of the left hemisphere was the brain's centre of speech (Beaton, 1985). The discovery soon followed that the motor centre for a limb on one side of the body was in the opposite half of the brain. The notion of hemispheric dominance was born.

The brain attracted attention as a neurological basis for hand preference. Theories of handedness and brain dominance relied heavily on explanations stemming from physiological asymmetry: unequal blood supply to the halves of the brain, differential hemispheric weight, asymmetrical brain convolutions, and differences in fissure length. Each received varying degrees of acceptance and skepticism. Even though no firm explanation for handedness could be offered, the wheels were set in motion for future avenues of neurological and physiological research.

Pathological evidence in the mid-1800's indicated that there was a higher incidence of disease and deformity on the left side of the body (Harris, 1980; Beaton, 1985). This was viewed as additional support for the superiority of the right side of the body and emerging concepts of left hemispheric dominance. It also laid the ground work for pathological explanations of left-handedness.

The asymmetry of handedness was applied to other motor areas and all senses in the late 19th Century. The idea of ocular and auditory dominance contributed to the growing complexity of extant handedness theories. Despite the fact that no data could be generated to support a correlation between ocular and manual dominance, ocular dominance research persisted into the 20th Century.

The 'arm length' theory appeared in the literature in the 20th Century. It was proposed that student handedness could be determined by measuring the length of the ulna in both arms. The longer of the two indicated hand dominance. Psychologists and educators took notice (Harris, 1980). After numerous measurements, Beeley (1919) questioned whether this was a reliable indicator of handedness.

Despite the problems and misleading paths of inquiry, patently incorrect theories fell by the wayside while those bearing some basis in fact endured. Most significantly, the rudimentary ideas of neurophysiological asymmetry and brain dominance opened the doors to a rich and complex field of research (Steinmetz, et al., 1991; Jordan, Patching and Thomas, 2003; Sibner, et al., 2002; Sainburg, 2002; Sainburg and Schaefer, 2004).

Positional Asymmetry

A French physiologist named Joseph Achille Comte studied the birth positions in 20,539 cases (Harris, 1980). The data accumulated suggested some link to hand preference. He found that in 96% of birth presentations the vertex of the newborn's skull appeared first. Of these, 17,226 were reported to have first or left occipito-anterior positions (the infant's head facing the mother's right) while 2,153 involved second or 'right' position presentations (the infant's head facing left). Comte proposed that birth presentation was a clue to the infant's intrauterine position.

He was unable to prove, however, that newborns appearing in the first and second birth positions definitely became right-and left-handed respectively. For this reason the 'birth presentation' theory was overlooked, although it did reappear three more times under other authors. Ultimately, Overstreet (1938) concluded that there was no correlation between handedness and prenatal position.

The importance of uterine orientation reemerged relative to twins. It was found that there was a higher incidence of sinistrality among dizygotic and monozygotic twins (Wilson and Jones, 1932). Researchers were not willing to discuss a direct relationship between fetal position and handedness phenomena though. It was emphasized that such a relationship deserved consideration and that attitude remained (Harris, 1980; Beaton, 1985).

Pathological Left-Handedness

Accepting any one of the physiological or social theories discussed already, many scientists went one step further to say that left-handedness was a manifestation of some brain disorder, personality pathology, or both. These models tended to be most interesting to study and yet most unfair to left-handers because they focused on negative characteristics (Harris, 1980).

Sinistrality has been the target of negative cultural, educational, linguistic, and religious traditions. It is, therefore, no wonder that scientific theories eventually emerged which held left-handedness, as a state of degeneracy, accountable for the development of criminality and antisocial behaviour. Geneticists viewed it as a recessive trait linked to aspects of diminished mental ability and moral excellence (Jordan, 1911).

In 1903, a noted Italian criminologist named Cesare Lombroso reported that the proportion of left-handers was higher among certain types of criminals than among soldiers (Beaton, 1985). An anatomical study of criminal heads led him to believe that normal individuals had greater development in their left hemisphere while the converse was true of criminals and deviants. Smith (1917) examined delinquents and children in American 'industrial schools' concluding that wickedness accompanies left-handedness. These conclusions were remarkable considering that the surveys of the time were unrepresentative (Harris, 1980).

Several early writers criticised this work, pointing out that left-handedness was not necessarily a stigma of inferiority. Two types of left-handedness were named (Satz, 1972): the atavistic or constitutional type was attributed to an inversion of normal cerebral asymmetry; the pathological kind manifested after a cerebral lesion, predominated in epileptics and delinquents (Jordon, 1911; Brewster, 1913). This classification system anticipated later thinking (Satz, 1972).

Burt, an educational psychologist, and Blau, a psychoanalyst, were very influential proponents of the pathological view. Left-handedness was associated with infantile psychoneurosis, stubbornness, disobedience, and insecurity. These theorists were undaunted by the fact that their clinical evidence did not support their contentions (Harris, 1980; Boake, et al., 1983; Beaton, 1985; Charlton, 1988).

Various cultures symbolically associate the left hand with feminine traits as well as evilness (Silverstein and Silverstein, 1977; Witelson and Pallie, 1973). This view was echoed in early anatomical writings, wherein left-handedness was linked with the female state and specific reproductive functions were thought to occur on the left side in the female body.

Even more extreme, left-handedness was regarded as an indicator of deviance and homosexuality in men (Barsley, 1966). Wilhelm Fliess, Sigmund Freud's closest friend outlined a theory of bisexuality which included bilateralism and left-handedness (Bonaparte, Freud, and Kris, 1954). Freud was interested in this notion, but felt that any direct association between sexual disturbance and criminality was doubtful and inapplicable. Considering the strange relationship Freud and Fliess had, it is difficult to imagine that they were capable of objective inquiry regarding this area of research.

Once left-handedness had been linked to homosexuality, it did not take long before emotional, artistic, and sensitive characteristics were associated with sinistrality. Considerable mention was made of Leonardo da Vinci and Michelangelo, both of whom were left-handed (Silverstein and Silverstein, 1977; Harris, 1980).

The attribution of cognitive deficiencies soon followed. Stuttering and reversed writing were reported to occur more frequently among sinistral individuals. This soon led to the idea that the motor centres for writing and speaking were intimately associated with the language centre in the human brain (Beaton, 1985). It was thought that natural left-handers, when forced to write with the right, could develop problems in speech and writing habits, including dyscriptia, dysgraphia and dyslexia. Reversal of hand use, accordingly, was believed to relieve stuttering. A link between language and handedness was made, and work in this area continues.

It was also believed that left-handers were deficient in spatial cognitive abilities, owing to the incidence of mirror writing and so forth. Again, Leonardo's famous mirror writing style was often cited (Silverstein and Silverstein, 1977; Harris, 1980). It was thought that mirror writing was a natural method for sinistrals because they would tend to write from right to left. Detractors of the theory that left-handers are deficient in spatial cognition and intelligence often cited Lewis Carroll, another left-hander, and Leonardo as examples to the contrary.

Despite all of the very damaging notions that developed over the years, some useful ideas emerged and into the research pathology of handedness continues (Michael, et al., 2005). Even though the question of forcing left-handers to write with their right persisted until the 1950's, more psychologists and pediatricians came to agree that coercion was ineffective and dangerous in education. Finally, the prejudices of sexuality and temperament dissipated under a wave of objective inquiry and clinical research throughout the medical, psychological and educational fields (Beaton, 1985; Harris, 1980).

Cultural Conditioning

It was as early as the 17th Century when 'nurturists' started rallying against the 'nativists' regarding the theoretical basis of hand preference. They were convinced that handedness did not depend on heredity or physiological asymmetries. Rather, they believed dextral predominance was strictly the result of learning and societal conditioning. Elements of their theories described below have lingered to this day.

In the 1880s, the importance of the child's position while being nursed or carried by the mother was held to have an influence on hand preference (Harris, 1980; Beaton, 1985). It was conjectured that, in most instances, a nurse would carry a child on her right arm, thus leaving the infant's right arm free to move and develop. The infant-holding theory had one immediate problem though. It was observed that mothers commonly carry their children in the left arm. This was confirmed by Burt (1937) through personal observation of 100 mothers, as well as a survey of artistic depictions of the Madonna and Child.

The warfare-shield theory, as described earlier, pointed to historical evidence that indicated dextrality was the norm because the heart side of the body needed protection. Critics of this theory cited the use of single-handed implements like the club and javelin. Shields were not employed with these weapons. Cultural one-handedness would have developed long before the advent of the shield, and another point emerged. If left-handers were more vulnerable by failing to protect the left their bodies, why did they survive (Silverstein and Silverstein, 1977; Harris, 1980)?

These theories received little attention in the 19th Century. Nurturists focussed on the actual hand preference of the human infant. Studies of babies and children were undertaken as sources of critical information both for and against the societal-conditioning view of handedness. Several researchers presented observations of their own children but drew no conclusions (Harris, 1980). The first truly experimental investigation was performed by James Baldwin (1890; 1894) using his daughter as a subject. He elicited unsymmetrical reaching behaviour by presenting objects just beyond her grasp. From the results, he concluded that his daughter had developed right-handedness under the pressure of muscular effort.

Similar investigations by others followed 15 years later. Their conclusions supported the premise that right-handedness was a normal part of physiological development, not a phenomenon controlled by training (Nice, 1918; Woolley, 1910).

These theories depended fundamentally on some sort of physiological explanation of handedness. However, in the 1920s the American scientific community shifted toward behaviourism under the influence of John Watson (Beaton,1985). His research showed no uniformity in hand use nor fixed differentiation of response in either hand until a societal influence impinged upon an individual's behaviour. Watson was at a loss to explain how society could have consisted of a predominantly right-handed population to begin with. The existence of sinistrals could not be accounted for as well.

Despite deficiencies in these behavioural and developmental theories, the effects of societal convention and learning were known to hold some importance in the development of individual handedness. It was becoming apparent that handedness was not a simple phenomenon. Several factors, including heredity, conditioning, and physiology, were contributing to each person's hand preference. The mechanism was simply not one-dimensional.

At the turn of the 20th Century, there was a movement afoot that disputed the naturalness of dextral preferences. It was proposed that ambidexterity could ensue from rational education which allowed or encouraged individuals to develop naturally (Harris, 1980). This curious educational movement promised equal acquisition of writing and other skills by both hands. One proponent even went so far as to claim that both hands could carry out separate tasks independently because the brain, having two hemispheres, could be regarded as a 'double organ', one capable of accommodating separate and distinct thinking processes simultaneously (Jackson, 1905).

The most dramatic claim made concerning the benefit of ambidextral training was the promise that the effects of unilateral brain injury would be prevented or ameliorated by two-handed training (Harris, 1980).

The biggest criticism of the ambidextral culture was its apparent disregard for all of the accumulated evidence showing handedness to be innate and rooted in brain physiology (Crichton-Browne, 1907). This movement eventually subsided, falling victim to its own exaggerated claims and the preponderance of many other criticisms. However, some later educators continued to promote the benefits of two-handedness that had been promised earlier (Harris, 1980).

Hand Posture in Writing

Of any asymmetrical activity undertaken in our society today, handwriting is used most frequently to distinguish sinistrals from dextrals because it is simple and obvious (Barsley, 1970). The attention paid to writing habits by psychologists stems from the classical traditions of education, the teaching of penmanship the right-handed way (Beaton, 1985). Now, fortunately, students may develop the writing hand of their choice without disciplinary repercussions. Aside from the obvious humanistic and educational benefits of this trend, there have been research benefits. Another clue to the mystery of lateralization in the brain has been revealed – this being hand posture, particularly in the writing habits of sinistrals.

Individuals not only differ in their choice of writing hand but also in writing posture. Some utilize the normal position, in which the hand and forearm are kept straight, while others use the hooked or inverted position, in which the wrist is kept bent (Beaton, 1985).

It was suggested that the hooked position in left-handers prevented smudged writing and allowed the writer to see more clearly what was being written. With this argument, it was predicted that there would be a higher incidence of hooked dextral Israeli writers than Americans because Hebrew script proceeds from right to left (Herron, 1980). A greater frequency of Israeli dextrals with the inverted hand posture was not found, but it was also discovered that the inverted left-hander was less abundant among Israeli writers than among Americans (Shanon, 1978). A cultural or learning effect was suggested. As well, recent investigations have indicated that the inverted writing posture is more common among males than among females (Coren and Porac, 1979), thus suggesting a genetic or physiological mechanism.

It is generally understood that motor control in the upper limbs is performed by the contralateral hemisphere. There is evidence indicating this is true for the fine movements carried out by the distal musculature of the fingers (Herron, 1980; Beaton, 1985). It has been suggested that hand posture can reveal what part of the brain is controlling an individual's writing actions.

Levy and Reid (1976) proposed that upright or normal handwriting postures indicate there is contralateral hemispheric control for language in its written forms. Conversely, inverted hand postures were deemed to signify ipsilateral cerebral control. Some controversy over this hypothesis was generated by physiological research into neural pathways.

Moscovitch and Smith (1979) interpreted the results of their research as indicating that the inverted and normal writing postures could be attributed to differences in visuo-motor rather than sensori-motor organization. However, there is ample evidence throughout the literature pointing.

out differences in fine-motor or sensori-motor control as an explanation for writing postures (Barsley, 1970; Herron, 1980; Parlow, 1978; Beaton, 1985), and throughout this research it generally has been found that, unlike dextrals, sinistrals with normal writing postures show an advantage for the right hand in finger flexion. This suggests that the differences in writing posture can be explained by sensori-motor organisation as originally hypothesized by Levy and Reid (1976).

Considering the complexity of the human brain, it may be discovered in future research that visuo-motor and sensori-motor factors are intricately organized in the determination of hand preference and writing control. Other more subtle elements may be discovered as well.

Genetics and Hereditynversus Environmental Theories

At the turn of the 20th Century, speculation regarding the genetic basis of handedness took root (Beeley, 1919; Harris, 1980). Even Darwin had addressed this issue using his own child as a case study. German researchers were the strongest proponents while others explicitly denied any link to genetics whatsoever.

Very few systematic genetic investigations were performed in those early years and the results were often unclear. Subsequent family surveys produced clearer results. Of particular note, numerous double left-handed matings giving rise to entire families of sinistral offspring were recorded.

In 1922, Jordan wrote with assurance that left handedness was clearly genetic, and that the incidence of sinistrality closely followed the rules of inheritance as they were understood at that time. Several others supported this view (Ramaley, 1913), but a strictly recessive model predicted that left-handed couples would always produce left-handed children, and this was not the case. Recognition of learning effects and a growing awareness of the complexity of genetic mechanisms presaged further investigation and controversy. The genetic mystery would not be solved by a simple dominant-recessive model.

Still, reports of left-handed families were compiled. In one remarkable case, two left-handed parents produced children, all preferring the left hand (Harris, 1980). Some family surveys had weak report reliability. Nevertheless, a genetic influence was definitely indicated even though the underlying system was not yet clear. There were also suggestions that the defining of handedness was not a straightforward undertaking. Assumption of a strictly dichotomous classification system was deemed to be possibly misleading (Beaton, 1985).

Even in the 1970s and 1980s the inheritance of handedness was disputed (Corballis, 1980). Levy and Nagylaki (1972) proposed a model that explained variations in handedness and cerebral lateralization in terms of Mendelian principles. This view was founded on a tradition of genetic models occupying most of the 20th Century. Such investigators as Trankell (1955), Rife (1940), and Ramaley (1913) were just three who held firmly to the position that handedness was solely attributable to heredity. They disregarded the accumulating evidence which suggested a learning effect.

The environmental position has been hotly contended as well (Collins, 1988). Dextrality was regarded as a learned response to a right-handed environmental bias. Hence, left-handedness was deemed a failure to learn, either through physical defect, faulty education, or 'emotional negativism.' This, essentially, had been the nurture side of the argument. One can quickly identify notions that resemble the dangerous and prejudiced ideas of earlier research. Despite these extreme views, it is generally held that there is a genetic influence (Corballis, 1980; Beaton, 1985).

Annett (1972) proposed a model that is a compromise between these opposing views and was generally regarded as the more plausible genetic explanation (Corballis, 1980). Two fundamental suppositions were made. First, unsystematic environmental influences are the cause of a large random component in the distribution of inter-manual differences. Second, most people inherit a 'right shift' factor, perhaps through a single gene, such that the mean distribution favours dextrality. Some people may lack this gene. Annett further conjectured that these individuals should favour either hand equally on unbiased tests. Proof was later furnished that the lack of a right shift is a recessive trait (Annett, 1974).

Subsequent research found fault with Annett's model and data, but it is widely accepted that a genetic factor may well explain the overall bias among humans toward right-handedness and the left-cerebral control of speech (Corballis, 1980). In answer to criticisms of previous work, Annett (1978) indicated that accidental variation is likely a major determinant of handedness, and dextral bias is induced by a genetic factor. The underlying genetic mechanisms are more complex. Current disagreement concerns the cause of left-handedness. Although Annett argued that some incidence of sinistrality could be explained in terms of a recessive trait, many believe there is insufficient evidence to support this notion (Corballis, 1980; Beaton, 1985). Many researchers held that environmental causes are at the root of sinistrality, but this notion garnered decreasing attention. According to Carter-Saltzman (1980), the results of a shared biological heritage, rather than sociological factors, are more significant in hand preference. More recent research revealed that the LRRTM1 gene appears to play a key role in determining which parts of the brain control specific functions, including the flip to left-handedness (Francks, at el., 2007).

Developmental Psychology and Learning Implications

The scientific dispute over whether handedness is a genetic, physiological, or environmental phenomenon continued. However, many of the old fallacies fell under a growing legacy of reliable and convincing research data.

It is now known that dextrality has some genetic basis while societal and environmental pressures influence left-handedness through learning effects. Currently, investigators recognize that gross-motor, upper-limb movements are contralaterally controlled. The neurological pathways for fine-motor or sensori-motor movements are being unravelled. Research supports the theory that the speech centres in the brain can be associated with the motor centres that control the dominant hand. It is known that there is a higher occurrence of sinistrals among twins and males in the human population. Credence is also given to the opinion that left-handedness can be a response to pathological factors in some cases. Important questions still remain unanswered.

Beyond the constructs of psychology and the mechanisms of genetics and physiology, handedness exists as a holistic phenomenon. It is a unique expression of an individual's connection to his or her environment and it has social and pedagogical implications.

As Tichy and Belacek (2009) and other researchers (Ramsay, 1980) discovered, handedness manifests in infants between seven and 13 months of age, and it is well established in 3-year-old children. Laterality appears to be stabilized by year ten. An investigation of the degree of correlation between handedness and physiological neocebellar extinction syndrome, confirmed that the motor cortex of the left hemisphere, in connection with the right cerebellar hemisphere, is responsible for cerebellar dominance and handedness. There has been evidence that handedness develops in the womb (Hepper and Shahidullah, 1990; 1991; Hepper, et al., 1998). Laterality, which appears to be stabilized in children by the age of 10, "appears to be a structurally arranged complex of physiological phenomena not quite dependent on one another" (Tichy and Belacek, 2009, p. 18). Data pertaining to cross-footedness indicated that neocerebral dominance correlates with hand dominance, which suggests that the learning of new asymmetrical or uni-manual skills will be governed by established hand dominance and brain laterality.

This, and similar research, provides a foundation for why it has been long understood that early forced learning relative to preferred handedness can have detrimental effects on an individual student's speech, reading and writing (Beaton, 1985; Clark, 1974). There may be other negative outcomes. This holds particular significance for modern educators, especially those concerned with language arts, and probably instructors of physical education and outdoor recreation (Clark, 1974; Grady, 1984).

The Challenge of Measuring Handedness

It can be a misleading oversimplification to determine whether one hand is superior over another based on individual respondents. Handedness is more complex than a simple binary attribution. The relationship of the right hand to the left depends on how the various digits are coordinated to execute different tasks in a finely programmed sequence of movements, and both hands can share complex tasks in varying ways (Herron, 1980; Beaton, 1985).

There are two fundamental questions faced by researchers. How should handedness be defined? How can it be reliably measured? This determination has been quite often arbitrary, which accounts for many of the contradictions throughout the handedness literature (Provins, 1967; Oldfield, 1971; Todor and Doane, 1977; Annett et al., 1979; Ransil and Schacter, 1994; Dragovic and Hammond, 2007), especially prior to 2000. Historically, people have been classified into three basic types: dextral, sinistral, and ambidextral – and more recently the terms mixed, inconsistent or shared handedness have been employed (Provins, 1967; Miller, 1971; Flowers, 1975, 1983; Steingruber, 1975; Briggs and Nebes, 1975; Bryden, 1977; Peters and Durding, 1978; Loo and Schneider, 1979; Peters, 1981). This simple classification does not account for the full range of manual asymmetry which can be observed. Handedness is more realistically modelled as a continuous distribution ranging from strongly right-handed to strongly left-handed (Annett, 1970; 1992; Peters and Durding,1978).

There are two distinguishable aspects of handedness that must be recognized in surveys: preference and skill. Numerous traditional techniques dominate this research. The Edinburgh Handedness Inventory has been employed extensively (Oldfield, 1971). Annett (1967) utilized a questionnaire that distinguished 12 behaviours or tasks. After analysing the responses from 2,321 subjects, Annett determined that there are at least 23 types of hand preference. It was then argued that handedness should not be regarded as a discrete variable. This inquiry was followed up using a peg-moving task (Annett, 1970). It was found that the degree of preference, as assessed by a questionnaire, correlated with the times taken by the two hands to place pegs into close-fitting holes. Conversely, Todor and Doane (1977) found a diminishing degree of correlation between left-handed manual preference and the difference in left-hand proficiency scores as task difficulty increased. However, it has been argued that the latter investigation produced a somewhat misleading conclusion (Beaton, 1985). By increasing task difficulty, the nature of the task is altered, and there is no reason to suppose that there is the same degree of symmetry between the hands regarding different components of movement control.

Using the Annett Hand Preference Questionnaire, Dragovic and Hammond (2007) found that 66% of those surveyed were consistently right-handed, 9.8% were consistently left-handed, 24.2% indicated inconsistent or mixed handedness. It was recommended that this questionnaire be updated with modern or relevant tasks. Other survey instruments and external methods of assessing brain laterality and uni-manual dexterity have included the Briggs-Nebes modified version of Annett's Handedness Inventory (Briggs and Nebes, 1975; Loo and Schneider, 1979), the Purdue Pegboard test of manual dexterity in conjunction with the Edinburgh Handedness Inventory (Verdino and Dingman, 1998), Bishop's reaching card test (Doyen and Carlier, 2002), and a multivariate approach using hand preference and hand performance measures (Annett, 1992; Corey and Hurley, 2001; Brown, et al., 2006)). The notion of continuously distributed handedness is widely accepted.

The assumption that laterality should be evaluated along a unidimensional continuum was later brought into question (Corey and Hurley, 2001). A lattice analysis was employed to determine if the structure of hand preference was equal for dextrals and sinistrals. Within the limits of a small sample space, right-handed behaviour appeared to be more global while nearly all left-handers exhibited distinct profiles.

Calvert (1998) discovered that, when performing an unskilled motor task, left-handers showed greater readiness to use the non-preferred hand than right-handers. Similarly, Crovitz and Zener (1962) reported that left-handers are less consistently sinistral in their manual preference than right-handers are dextral. This is a problem when classifying left- and right-handed groups. Bryden (1977) found that dextrals show a strong preference for the right hand when tested objectively, but many who describe themselves as left-handed will in fact preferentially use the right hand for a number of activities. Left-handers vary more in their reporting of hand use than dextrals, and the within-subject consistency in hand use for particular tasks among sinistrals is also lower. This pointed out that the criteria for surveying left-handers should be more universal and better defined. Calvert (1998), employing a behavioural continuum, found that left-handers showed greater readiness to use the non-preferred hand than right-handers when performing an unskilled task.

Two types of movement were distinguished by Flowers in 1975. 'Ballistic' hand movements are made without feedback (like throwing a ball) while 'corrective' motions require a feedback loop to monitor and modify hand motions (like carrying a spoon of soup up to the mouth). It was found that in strongly lateralized individuals – either dextrals or sinistrals – the preferred hand performed better than the non-preferred hand when it came to corrective movements. 'Ambilateral' or ambidextrous individuals showed poor control in the preferred hand without any compensatory increase in the skill of the non-preferred hand. Flowers (1975, 1983) also found that individuals having a manual preference that was not so distinct showed superior skill in the non-preferred hand. Hence, hand skill depends on the degree of manual preference and whether the required task is ballistic or corrective. Further, Steehuis and Bryden (1989) identified four types of handedness: skilled actions, reaching actions, power actions and bimanual actions.

Hand differences also depend upon the type of movement and its complexity (Steingruber, 1975; Provins, 1967; Peters, 1981). Practice seems to diminish the difference in skill level between the hands for certain tasks while the asymmetry remains constant for others. This was investigated by Annett, Hudson and Turner in 1979. It was found that the non-preferred hand was slower and more variable during the aiming phases of tasks (corrective movements).

Nakamura and Saito (1974) recorded electrical measurements of muscle contractions. Reaction times were faster for the preferred hand in supination but the non-preferred hand was quicker in flexion. This led them to believe that the two movements are controlled separately in the brain. It has been found that flexion of digits was carried out more quickly and with greater precision by left-hand fingers in people preferring the right hand (Kimura and Vanderwolf, 1970; Parlow, 1978). The relationship between the individual fingers is quite subtle and this further complicates the determination of skill differences between the right and left hands.

Hence, investigators are faced with the task of measuring handedness by degrees through examinations of hand skill and preference as separate characteristics. Types of skill, like corrective and ballistic, must be distinguished. The aim is to render more reliable conclusions by applying universal definitions and criterion cutoffs to data acquired through questionnaires and direct observations.

Recent Research

As noted, scientists from a wide range of disciplines – notably psychology, psychiatry, neurology, anatomy, and biology – have been investigating laterality differences in humans, and other species. Researchers in education have devoted some effort to the question of handedness. Sociology, anthropology, primate research, and comparative anatomy studies also contributed to evolving perspectives. Over the last half century, many studies on this subject have been published, only a few of which have been briefly described herein.

Current theories have been built upon the sounder ideas that have endured from early investigations and speculation. Considering the complexity of the human brain, it may be discovered in future research that visuo-motor and sensori-motor factors are intricately organized in the determination of hand preference, skill and writing control. Other more subtle elements may be discovered as well.

The scientific discussion pertaining to genetic, physiological, and environmental factors will continue, and old fallacies have fallen under a legacy of reliable and convincing research data. It is now known that dextrality has a neuroanatomical and genetic basis while societal and environmental pressures influence handedness through learning effects.

Beyond the constructs of psychology and the mechanisms of genetics and physiology, handedness exists as a holistic phenomenon. It is a unique expression of an individual's connection to his or her environment and it has social and pedagogical implications. The challenge for investigators has been and will continue to be associated with how to define and assess handedness.

References

Annett, M. (1967). The binomial distribution of right, mixed and left handers. *Quarterly Journal of Experimental Psychology,* 19, 327-334.

Annett, M. (1970). A classification of hand preference by association analysis. *British Journal of Psychology,* 61 (3), 303-321.

Annett, M. (1972). The distribution of manual asymmetry. *British Journal of Psychology,* 63, 343-358.

Annett, M. (1973). Handedness in families. *Annals of Human Genetics,* 37 (1), 93-105.

Annett, M. (1974). Handedness in the children of two left-handed parents. *British Journal of Psychology, 65*, 129-131.

Annett, M. (1978). Genetic and nongenetic influences on handedness. *Behavior Genetics,* 8 (3), 227-249.

Annett, J., Annett, M., Hudson, P.T.W., and Turner, A. (1979). The control of movements in the preferred and non-preferred hands. *Quarterly Journal of Experimental Psychology,* 31, 641-652.

Annett M. (1992). Five tests of hand skill. *Cortex,* 28, 583-600.

Baldwin, J. (1890). Origin of right or left handedness. *Science,* 16, 2, 47-248.

Baldwin, J. (1894). The origin of right-handedness. *Popular Science Monthly,* 44, 606-615.

Balter, Michael. (2009). The origins of handedness, *The Science of Origins. American Association for the Advancement of Science.* Posted August 18, 2009 at http://sciencemag.org/origins/2009/08/the-origins-of-handedness.html

Barsley, M. (1966). T*he Other Hand: An Investigation Into the Sinister History of Left-handedness.* New York: Hawthorn.

Barsley, M. (1970). *Left-handed Man in a Right-handed World.* London, Great Britain: Pitman Publishing.

Beaton, A. (1985). *Left Side, Right Side.* New Haven, Connecticut: Yale University Press.

Beck, L.F. (1936). Manual skills and the measurement of handedness. The *Journal of Psychology,* 2, 259-272.

Beeley, A. L. (1919). Left-handedness. *American Journal of Physical Anthropology,* 2, 389-400.

Boake, C., Salmon, P. G., and Carbone, G. (1983). Torque, lateral preference, and cognitive ability in primary-grade children. *Journal of Abnormal Child Psychology,* 11 (1), 77-83

Bonaparte, M., Freud, A., Kris, E. (Eds.) (1954). *The Origins of Psychoanalysis: Letters to Wilhelm Fliess, Drafts, and Notes, 1887-1902 by Sigmund Freud.* New York: Basic Books.

Briggs, G. G., Nebes, R. D. Patterns of hand preference in a student populations. *Cortex,* 11 (3),230-8.

Brewster, E. T. (1913). The ways of the left hand. *McClure's Magazine,* 41 (June), 168-183.

Briggs, G.G., Nebes, R.D. (1975). Patterns of hand preference in a student population, *Cortex,* 11(3): 230-238.

Brown, S., Roy, E., Rohr, L., and Bryden, P. (2006). Using hand performance measures to predict handedness. *Laterality: Asymmetries of Body, Brain, and Cognition,* 11 (1), 1-14.

Bryden, M. P. (1977). Measuring handedness with questionnaires. *Neuropsychologia,* 15, 617-624.

Buchanan, A. (1862). Mechanical theory of the preponderance of the right hand of the left; or, more generally, of the limbs of the right side over the left side of the body. *Proceedings of the . Philosophical Society of Glasgow,* 5, 142-107.

Burt, C. (1937). *The Backward Child.* London, England: University of London Press.

Calvert G. A. (1998). Quantifying hand preference using a behavioural continuum. *Laterality: Asymmetries of Body, Brain and Cognition,* 3 (3), 255-268.

Carter-Saltzman, L. (1980). Biological and sociocultural effects on handedness: comparison between biological and adoptive families. *Science,* 209 (4462), 1263-1265

Casey, M. B., Brabeck, M.M., and Ludlow, L. H. (1986). Familial handedness and its relation to spatial ability following strategy instructions. I*ntelligence*, 10, 389-406.

Chamberlain, H. D. (1928). The inheritance of left-handedness. *Journal of Heredity,* 19, 557-559.

Charlton, S. (1988). Torque and cerebral laterlization: a questionable link. *International Journal of Neuroscience,* 43 (1-2), 15-19.

Clark, M.M. (1974). *Teaching Left-Handed Children.* London, England: University of London Press Ltd.

Collins, R. L. (1988). Observational learning of a left right asymmetry by mice (Mus musculus). *Journal of Comparative Psychology,* 102, 222-224.

Corballis, M.C. (1980). *Is left-handedness genetically determined?* In J. Herron (Ed.), *Neuropsychology of Left-handedness* (pp. 159-176). New York: Academic Press.

Coren, S. and Porac, C. (1979). Normative data on hand position during writing. *Coretex,* 15, 679-682.

Corey D. M., Hurley M.M., and Foundas A. L. (2001). Right and left handedness defined: a multivariate approach using hand preference and hand performance measures. *Neuropsychiatry, Neuropsychology and Behavioral Neurology,* 14 (3),144-52.

Crichton-Browne, J. (1907). Dexterity and the bend sinister. *Proceedings of the Royal Institution of Great Britain,* 18, 623-652.

Crovitz, H. and Zener, K. (1962). A group test for assessing hand-and-eye dominance. *American Journal of Psychology,* 75, 271-276.

Dragovic M, Hammond G. A classification of handedness using the Annett hand preference questionnaire. *British Journal of Psychology*, 98 (3), 375-87.

Doyen, A. L., and Carlier. M. (2001). Measuring handedness: a validation study of Bishop's reaching card test. *Laterality: Asymmetries of Body, Brain, and Cognition,* 7 (2), 115-130.

Doyen, A. L., Duquenne, V., Nuques, S., and Carlier, M. (2004). What can be learned from a lattice analysis of a laterality questionnaire? *Behavior Genetics,* 31 (2), 193-207.

Flowers, K. (1975). Handedness and controlled movement. *British Journal of Psychology,* 66 (1), 39-52.

Flowers, K. (1983). Manual performance asymmetries and motor control processes: subject-generated changes in response parameters. *Human Movement Science,* 2 (4)271-277.

Francks, C., Margawa, S., Laurén, J., Abrahams, B.S., Velayos-Baeza, A., Meland, S.E., Colella, S., Groszer, M., MaAuley, E.Z., et al. (2007). LRRTM1 on chromosome 2p12 is a maternally suppressed gene that is associated paternally with handedness and schizophrenia, *Journal of Molecular Psychiatry,* 12 (12), 1129-1139.

Hannaford, C. (2005). *Smart Moves: Why Learning is Not All in Your Head.* Salt Lake City: Great River Books.

Harris, L. J. (1980). Left-handedness: early theories, facts, and fancies. In Herron, J. (Ed.), *Neuropsychology of Left-handedness* (pp. 3-78). New York: Academic Press.

Hartlage, L. C., and Gage, R. (1997). Unimanual performance as a measure of laterality. *Neuropsychology Review,* 7 (3), 143-156.

Hepper, P. G., McCartney, G.R., and Shannon, E.A. (1998). Lateralized behaviour in first trimester human fetuses. *Neuropsychologia* 36, 531-534.

Herron, Jeannine (Ed.). (1980). *Neuropsychology of Left-handedness.* New York: Academic Press.

Herzfeld, C, and Lestel, D. (2006). Knot tying in great apes: etho-ethnology of an unusual tool behavior. *Social Science Information,* 44 (4) 621-653.

Hopkins, W. D., Dunham, L., Cantalupo, C., and Taglialatela, J. (2007). The association between handedness, brain asymmetry and corpus callosum size in chimpanzees (Pan troglodytes). *Cerebral Cortex,* 17 (8), 1757-1765.

Hopkins, W. D., and Russell, J. L. (2004). Further evidence of a right hand advantage in motor skills by chimpanzees (Pan troglodytes), *Neuropsychologia,* 42 (7), 2004, 990-996.

Jackson, J. (1905). *Ambidexterity or Two-handedness and Two-brainedness.* London, England: Kegan Paul, Trench, Trubner and Co., Ltd.

Jordan, H. E. (1911). The inheritance of left-handedness. *American Breeder's Magazine, 2*, 19-28; 113-124.

Jordan, H. E. (1922). The crime against left-handedness. *Good Health,* 57, 378-383.

Jordan, T. R., Patching, G. R. (2003). Assessing the role of hemispheric specialisation, serial-position processing, and retinal eccentricity in lateralised word recognition, *Cognitive Neuropsychology*, 2003, 20 (1), 49-71.

Kimura, D. and Vanderwolf, C.H. (1970). The relation between hand preference and the performance of individual finger movements by left and right hands. *Brain,* 93, 769-774.

Laska, M. (1996). Manual laterality in spider monkeys (Ateles geoffroyi) solving visual and tactually guided food-reaching tasks. *Cortex* 32 (4), 717-726.

Levy, J. and Nagylaki, T. (1972). A model for genetics of the hand. *Genetics,* 72, 117-128.

Levy, J. and Reid, M. L. (1976) Variations in writing posture and cerebral organization. *Science,* 194, 337-339.

Loo, R., and Schneider, R. (1979). An evaluation of the Briggs-Nebes modified version of Annett's handedness inventory. *Cortex,* 15 (4), 683-686.

McCartney, G. R., and Hepper, P.G. (1999). Development of laterized behaviour in the human fetus from 12-27 weeks' gestation. Developmental Medicine and *Child Neurology,* 41, 83-86

Miller, E. (1971). Handedness and the pattern of human ability. *British Journal of Psychology,* 7, 19-48.

Moscovitch. M., and Smith, L.C. (1979). Differences in neural organisation between individuals with inverted and non-inverted handwriting postures. *Science,* 205, 710-712.

Nakamura, R., and Saito, H. (1974). Preferred hand and reaction time in different movement patterns. *Perceptual and Motor Skills,* 39, 1275-1281.

Netley, C. (1988). Relationships between hemispheric lateralization, sex hormones, quality of parenting and adjustment in 47, XXY males prior to puberty. *Journal of Child Psychology and Psychiatry,* 29 (3), 282-287.

Nice, M.M. (1918). Ambidexterity and delayed speech development. *Pedagogical Seminary,* 25, 141-162.

Oldfield, R. C. (1971) The assessment of handedness: the Edinburgh inventory. *Neuropsychologia*, 9, 97-113.

Olson, D. R. (1970). *Cognitive Development: The Child's Acquisition of Diagonality.* New York: Academic Press.

Overstreet, R. (1938). An investigation of prenatal position and handedness. *Psychological Bulletin,* 35, 520-521.

Parlow, S. (1978). Differential finger movements and hand preference. *Cortex,* 14, 608-611.

Peters, M. (1981). Handedness effect of prolonged practice on between hand performance differences. *Neuropsychologia,* 19, 570-590.

Peters, M. and Durding, B. M. (1978). Handedness measured by finger tapping: a continuous variable. *Canadian Journal of Psychology,* 32, 257-261.

Provins, K. A. (1967). Motor skills, handedness and behaviour. *Australian Journal of Psycholoqy,* 19, 137-150.

Ramaley, F. (1913). Inheritance of left-handedness. *American Naturalist,* 47, 730-738.

Ramsay, D. S. (1980). Onset of unimanual handedness in infants. *Infant Behaviour and Development, 3*, 377-385.

Ransil, B. J., Schachter, S.C. (1994). Test-re test reliability of the Edinburgh Handedness Inventory and global handedness preference measurements, and their correlation. *Perceptual and Motor Skills,* 79 (1), 1355-1372.

Rife, D. C. (1940). Handedness, with special reference to twins. *Genetics,* 25, 178-186.

Sainburg, R. L. (2002). Evidence for dynamic-dominance hypothesis of handedness. *Experimental Brain Research*, 142, 241-258, 2002.

Sainburg, R. L., and Schaefer, S. Y. (2004). Interlimb differences in control of movement extent. *Journal of Neurophysiology,* 92, 1374-1383.

Satz, P. (1972). Pathological left-handedness: An explanatory model. *Cortex,* 8, 121-135.

Shanon, B. (1978). Writing positions in Americans and Israelis. Neuro-psychologia, *16, 587-591.*

Schulter-Ellis, F.P. (1980). Evidence of handedness on documented skeletons. *Journal of Forensic Sciences,* 25 (3), 624-630.

Siebner, H. R., Limmer, C., Peinemann, A., Drzezga, A., Bloem, B. R., Schwaiger, M., and Conrad, B. (2002). Long-term consequences of switching handedness: a positron emission tomography study on handwriting in "converted" left-handers. *The Journal of Neuroscience,* 22 (7), 2816-2825.

Silverstein, A. and Silverstein, V.B. (1977). *The Left-Hander's World.* Chicago: Follet Publishing.

Smith, L. G. (1917). A brief survey of right- and left-handedness. *Pedagogical Seminary,* 24, 19-35.

Steenhuis, R. E., and Bryden, M. P. (1989). Different dimensions of hand preference that relate to skilled and unskilled activities. *Cortex,* 25 (2), 289-304.

Steingruber, H.J. (1975). Handedness as a function of test complexity. *Perceptual and Motor Skills,* 40, 263-266.

Steinmetz, H., Volkmann, J., Jäncke, L., and Freund, H.J. (1991). Anatomical left-right asymmetry of language-related temporal cortex is different in left- and right-handers, *Anals of Neurology,* 29 (3), 315-319.

Sumners, D. W. (1987). The role of knot theory in DNA research. In McCory, C. and Shifrin, T. (Eds.), Geometry and Topology: Manifolds, Varieties and Knots. *Lecture Notes in Pure and Applied Mathematics,* 105, 297-318, New York: Dekker.

Sun, T., and Alsh, C. A. (2006). Molecular level brain asymmetry. *Nature Reviews Neurosceince,* 7, 655-662.

Tichy, J., and Belacek, J. (2009). Laterality in children: cerebellar dominance, handedness, footedness and hair whorl. *Activitas Nervosa Superior Rediviva,* 51, (1-2), 9-20.

Todor, J. I., and Doane, T. (1977). Handedness classification: preference versus proficiency. *Perceptual and Motor Skills,* 45, 1041-1041.

Trankell, A. (1955). Aspects of genetics in psychology. *American Journal of Human Genetics,* 7, 264-276.

Tuthill, H. (1994). *Individualization: Principles and Procedures in Criminalistics.* Salem, Oregon: Lightning Powder Company, Inc.

Uomini, N. T. (2009). The prehistory of handedness: archeological data and comparative ethology. *Journal of Human Evolution,* 57 (4), 411-419.

Verdino M, Dingman, S. (1998). Two measures of laterality in handedness: the Edinburgh Handedness Inventory and the Purdue Pegboard Test of manual dexterity. *Perceptual and Motor Skills,* 86 (20), 476-8.

Witelson, S. F., and Pallie, W. (1973). Left hemisphere specialization for language in the newborn: neuroanatomical evidence of asymmetry. *Brain,* 96, 641-646.

Woolley, H. T. (1910). The development of right-handedness in a normal infant. *Psychological Review,* 17, 37-41.

In: Handedness: Theories, Genetics and Psychology ISBN: 978-1-61470-502-4
Editors: J. Dunham and T. Davenport

Chapter III

Manual Laterality and Hemispheric Specialization for Language: A Review from Ancient Theories to Current Facts

Georges Dellatolas*[*], *Françoise Morange-Majoux* and *Christelle Lemoine
University Paris Descartes, Laboratory of Cognitive Psychology and Neuropsychology, FRE 3292 CNRS

Abstract

The aim of this article is to describe ancient and modern theories of human laterality based on recent data on manual and cerebral specialization. Manual specialization and handedness are distinct manifestations of manual laterality. Handedness results from genetic, environmental, pathological, and activity-related factors, and their interactions. Manual specialization is a more direct manifestation of cerebral specialization than handedness. In

[*] Corresponding author: Université Paris Descartes, Institut de Psychologie, Laboratoire de Psychologie et Neuropsychologie Cognitives, FRE 3292 CNRS, 71, avenue Edouard Vaillant, 92774, Boulogne-Billancourt. Tel. 01 55 20 58 17. Fax. 01 55 20 59 85. Email : georges.dellatolas@parisdescartes.fr.

young infants and in nonhuman primates, most of researches have demonstrated a manual specialization. Questions concerning measurement, uni- or multidimensionality, plasticity and activity-related factors, sex differences, or age effect, are common for the two domains, manual laterality and cerebral specialization, illustrating the strong link between manual gestures and language.

Keywords: Handedness, language, manual specialization, hemispheric specialization.

Introduction

Aristote thought that right-handedness was "natural", written into the body, whereas Plato thought that symmetry was natural and right-handedness a consequence of education (cited by Hécaen, 1984). This old debate continues presently, some people considering handedness as a fixed biologically determined characteristic of an individual, and others insisting on handedness plasticity and possibility of change. If Plato is right, education would be considered as repressive and even as creating a mutilation, as Reade (1878) claimed. In the USA, an ambidextrous society appeared at the beginning of the 20th century, based on the idea that the training of the two hands of an individual to do simultaneously two different thinks would double his/her thinking capacity (Jackson, 1905). On the contrary, if Aristote is right, left-handedness would be considered as atypical and even abnormal. The association of left-handedness with an accident or an handicap seems logical in some cases, simply due to the fact that most humans are right-handers. For instance, among people with only one hand (left or right) the proportion of left-handers is expected to be 50% instead of about 10% in the general population. Even in the absence of such an evident cause of left-handedness, it can be supposed nevertheless that all left-handers have some dysfunction of their left cerebral hemisphere (Bakan, 1990; Coren and Searlemann, 1990).

After the discovery of an hemispheric specialization for language by Broca (1861, 1865), who claimed that « we speak with the left hemisphere », handedness was considered as one manifestation of cerebral laterality. The dominant idea, adopted by Broca, was an innate hemispheric specialization having as one of its consequences right-handedness. However, the opposite idea, i.e., right-handedness determining left hemisphere language specialization, was also present at the end of the 19th century (Buzzard, 1882). In our days, Broca's model dominates, and arguments in favor come for instance from studies showing anatomical hemispheric asymmetries (e.g., Geschwind and Levitsky, 1968) or left hemispheric specialization for language in babies (Dehaene-Lambertz, Dehaene and Hertz-Pannier, 2002; Dubois, Hertz-Pannier, Cachia, Mangin, Le Bihan and Dehaene-Lambertz, 2009). Nevertheless, there are also recent data in favor of Bruzzard's idea, that is: hand activity influences hemispheric specialization for language: subjects who lost their right hand in childhood have presented aphasia after right hemisphere stroke in adulthood (Hécaen, 1984); cerebral palsy with right hemiplegia from infancy increases the probability of right hemisphere dominance for language (Rey, Dellatolas, Bancaud and Talairach, 1988); obstetric brachial plexus injury creating sever right hand dysfunction influence right speech dominance (Auer, Pinter, Kovacs, Kalmar, Nagy, Horvath, Koszo, Kotek, Perlaki, Koves, Kalman, Komoly, Schwarcz, Woermann and Janszky, 2009); finally, stimulation of the activity of the left hand in right hemiplegic subjects with aphasia was proposed for the reeducation of aphasia with the idea that such activity influence right hemisphere involvement in language (Crosson, 2008).

Geschwind and Galaburda's (1985) theory of cerebral lateralization postulates that "standard dominance" in humans (i.e., right-handedness and left hemisphere specialization for language) is determined by genetic factors and "atypical dominance" by hormonal factors, and in particular testosterone, acting in utero. In addition, associations of atypical dominance (e.g., left-handedness) with various diseases and specific cognitive profiles were suggested (Geschwind and Behan, 1982). Many studies continue to report arguments in favor or against this theory. For instance, Lust, Geuze, van de Beek, Cohen-Kettenis, Groothuis and Bouma (2009), report an association of testosterone level in utero and language lateralization at 6 years of age, but Mercure, Ashwin, Dick, Halit, Auyeung, Baron-Cohen and Johnson (2009) did not observe a testosterone effect on lateralization in boys.

The role of *in utero* factors on lateralization is an old idea. Joseph-Achille Comte (1828) claimed that handedness is determined by the position of the foetus, and Leurat and Gratiolet (1857) wrote that the two cerebral hemispheres develop with different timing. More recently Turkewitz (1988) adopts this latter idea to explain left-hemispheric specialization for language by the acoustic environment of the foetus: the human foetus perceives speech sounds at the end of gestation, but perceives only noise (e.g., mother's heart and gastro-intestinal noises) earlier in gestation; as the right temporal cortex matures earlier than the left, there will be right dominance for the treatment of noises and left dominance for the treatment of speech. Previc (1991) explains hemispheric specialization by the asymmetry of acoustic and vestibular afferences in utero: the former, due to asymmetrical craniofacial development generate a right ear advantage and left hemisphere dominance for speech, the latter due to the position of the foetus in utero, influence right hemisphere visuo-spatial dominance and right-handedness.

As human lateralization includes both manual activity and language, a general question is: what is the link between hand and language? There is evidence that this link is strong. In the deaf, communication may rely mainly or exclusively on hand gestures, and sign language seems to depend on the same areas of the cerebral cortex as oral language (Campbell, MacSweeney and Waters, 2008). Spontaneous gestures in children aged 2 to 5 years with deafness appear to have the same structure as oral language (Goldin-Meadow, Mylander and Butcher C, 1995; Goldin-Meadow and Mylandre, 1998). Gestures accompanying speech in hearing subjects are asymmetrical (Saucier and Elias, 2001), and may act as facilitating the thinking of the speaking subject (Goldin-Meadow, 1999), without having necessarily a communication role (e.g., blind subjects make the same gestures during communication with other blind subjects: Iverson and Goldin-Meadow, 1998). In young children gestures precede and prepare language development. Pointing gestures at 18 months may transform in sentence (mi-verbal mi-gesture), a word pronounced in isolation, for instance a verb (Iverson and Goldin-Meadow, 2005) and gesture analysis at 18 months of age could predict language development at 3 years (Rowe and Goldin-Meadow, 2009). Finally, according to Corballis' (1998, 2002, 2009) theory of evolution of language, gestures are at the origin of human language.

In the following we discuss the association of manual laterality with hemispheric specialization for language: classical studies of the link between handedness and language laterality; methodological problems related to the definition and measurement of lateralities ; gender differences ; developmental aspects ; pathology-related issues.

I. Exploring the Relation between Handedness and Hemispheric Specialization for Language

What proportion of right- and left-handers shows left or right hemisphere dominance for language? A classical method for answering this question is the clinical observation of the effect of unilateral cerebral lesions in subjects with known handedness. For instance, Hécaen and Ajuriaguerra (1963) examined 309 right-handed patients (173 with left hemisphere and 136 with right hemisphere lesion) and 59 left-handed patients (37 LH, 22 RH) and concluded that aphasia is more frequent but less severe in left-handers due to reduced hemispheric specialization for language. The temporary inactivation of one hemisphere by injection of Amobarbital in one carotid artery (Wada and Rasmussen, 1960) is another classical method exploring hemispheric specialization for language in subjects who are candidates for a neurosurgical treatment, often for epilepsy: the subject may or may not present aphasia during this inactivation. Using this method in 262 subjects with epilepsy but "without early left hemisphere lesion" Rasmussen and Milner (1977) reported 96% left- and 4% right-hemisphere dominance for language in right-handers (n=140) and 70% left-, 15% bilateral, 15% right hemisphere dominance in non-right-handers (i.e. left-handers and subjects with mixed preference for handedness). This report is always cited as a reference for the link between handedness and cerebral laterality for language. A recent report using the same method in the same population (174 epilepsy surgery candidates) gives markedly different results in non-right-handers: frequency of atypical (i.e. non-left) language dominance was 9% in strong right-handers, 46% in ambidextrous, and 69% in strong left-handers.

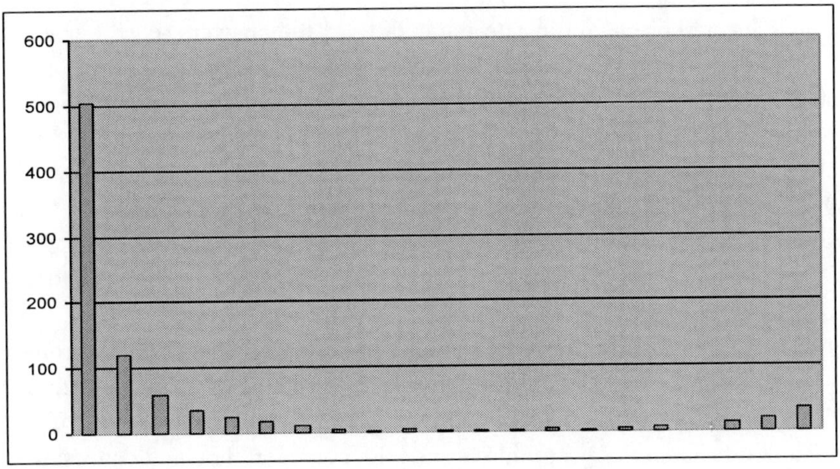

Figure 1. Typical asymmetrical U-shaped distribution of handedness score. In this example 882 adults were asked to indicate the hand used for 10 familiar unimanual activities. Each answer was coded 0 for « right hand », 1 for « both hands », and 2 for « left hand ». The score varies from 0 (strong right handedness to 20 strong left-handedness).

Modern investigations exploring language laterality use methods easier to apply than systematic clinical observation of right- and left-handed patients with unilateral brain lesions, and less invasive than the Wada test, applicable in healthy subjects (fMRI, PET, MEG, transcranial functional Doppler, etc.). However, it remains difficult to give a brief summary of the results of all these studies concerning the relation between manual laterality and language laterality. We suggest in the following some reasons explaining this difficulty.

II. Methodological Issues: Definition and Assessment of Handedness, Manual Specialization, and Cerebral Specialization

In adults, the definition and measurement of handedness is based most often on questionnaires (See Olfield, 1971), where subjects have to answer which hand they use for a variable number of activities, from one to 20 or more. Handedness questionnaires have generally an unifactorial structure, which means that answers at all items are strongly inter-correlated, without evidence of more that one clusters. The first component at Principal Component Analysis explains most of the variance and Cronbach's alpha is high. This justifies the calculation of only one handedness score summing up the coding of the answers (e.g., 1=right hand, 2=two hands, 3=left hand; or 1=always right hand, 2=right more than left, 3=equal, 4=left more than right, 5=always right). The distribution of the handedness score in the population is asymmetrical U-shaped (Figure 1). In young children, questionnaires are not well-adapted, and handedness is often assessed using demonstration tasks, which lead to the same asymmetric U-shaped distributions in the population (Dellatolas, De Agostini, Jallon, Poncet, Rey, and Lellouch, 1988; Curt, Mesbah, Lellouch and Dellatolas, 1997; Dellatolas et Lazaratou, 1989).

Based on this distribution, it is possible to define two handedness groups (e.g, right-handers=more right than left answers, left-handers=more left than right answers), to define more than two groups (e.g., four or five: strong and weak right- and left-handers, $\pm$ ambidextrous), to consider the handedness score as continuous, or to calculate an always positive or equal to zero degree of handedness (i.e. distance from the point where the number of right answers equal the number of left answers). It can be shown that the definition of right- and left-handers adopting the answers majority criterion given above is relatively robust (i.e., fairly independent of the number of items or the number of answer modalities at each item), contrary to the definition for strong/weak handedness groups, which is strongly dependent on the specific questionnaire used.

Table 1 shows the proportion of left-handers we observed in different countries. This proportion was slightly lower in the south of Europe and in African countries than in France (8-10%) or in USA and England (about 10%) (Halpern and Coren, 1988). In India, the proportion of left-handed children (3.2%) was 3 times lower than in France (9.6%) (Singh, Manjary and Dellatolas, 2001). Both genetic and environmental factors could explain these differences.

In some instances, more than one handedness components might appear (e.g., when some specific activities are under strong social pressure against the use of one hand; when the questionnaire includes bimanual or unfamiliar activities or repetitions of almost the same item such as pick-up different objects; etc.). In this case, a subject can be left-hander according to the first handedness component but right-hander according to the second (e.g. a left-hander who uses his right hand for writing).

Table 1. Frequency of left-handedness observed in different countries

	N	% left-handed
France	2367	9.3
Greece	703	6.4
Spain	737	6.6
Italy	710	7.2
Algeria	682	5.7
Soudan	759	5.0

Table 2. Proportion of left-handers writing with their left hand. Pooled data from France, Italy, Spain, and Greece (Dellatolas et al., 1991)

Age (in 1988)	N left-handers	% left-hand writing
15-19	44	82
20-24	52	63
25-29	72	54
30-34	76	54
35-39	46	39
40-49	47	11
≥50	28	18

Social pressure against the use of one hand might be global, reducing for instance the proportion of left-handers, or specific, concerning only particular activities, such as writing or "unclean" hand usage. Specific pressure are easier to show, because they appear as secondary handedness components not congruent with overall handedness, for instance as right-hand writing in a left-hander or as left-hand usage to clean his/her nose in a right-hander. The former was clearly observed in France and South-European countries (Dellatolas and Lazaratou, 1989), with older (but not younger) left-handers being right-hand writers (table 2); the latter was observed in Soudan, where 70% of the students declared use their left-hand to clean their nose (De Agostini, Hassan Khamis, Ahui and Dellatolas, 1997).

The above considerations partly explain why handedness studies often lead to contradictory findings. In particular, the dichotomy strong right-handers versus non-strong right-handers will vary from one study to the other according to the tool used to assess handedness.

Furthermore, some authors might use the term handedness as synonymous of functional asymmetry of the hands in general, which includes not only manual preference (i.e., questionnaire or demonstration based, as above) but also all aspects of manual specialization.

The latter will be defined here as the advantage of one hand over the other at different tasks assessing manual skill. For instance, we can measure the performance of the right hand (R) and of the left-hand (L) at a task like the Peg-moving, then calculate a the relative difference (R-L)/(R+L), which is often called Laterality Index (LI). The "right shift theory" of Annett (2002) is based on this index at the Peg-moving task. Such an index has generally a bell-shaped distribution (or close to it) in the general population, contrary to the U-shaped distribution of manual preference (Figure 2). This suffices to show that manual preference and manual specialization as defined above are quite different phenomena, and also suggests snow-ball effects, possibly activity-dependent, on the former but not necessarily on the latter. It is clear that LI depends on the specific task used to assess hand skill. LI and MP are generally correlated, however the degree of this correlation may be task-dependent. For instance, using some tasks, it is possible to find two bell-shaped distributions, one corresponding to right-handers and the other to left-handers; but using other tasks, only one bell-shaped distribution appears, and although the mean LI differs significantly between right- and left-handers (according to manual preference questionnaires), some right-handers show left hand advantage and some left-handers right-hand advantage (De Agostini, Paré, Goudot, and Dellatolas, 1992; Curt, Maccario and Dellatolas, 1992).

Is manual specialization, as defined above, an unidimensional trait? It remains difficult to answer this question, because there are not enough studies in the general population proposing numerous manual tasks assessing all aspects of manual skill, with calculation of all task-specific LIs and analysis of their correlation matrix. However, a recent study deals with this question, but focusing on hemispheric specialization instead of manual specialization: is hemispheric specialization an unidimensional phenomenon or is it better to consider it as including more than one dimension? (Whitehouse and Bishop, 2009). In the first case right hemisphere visuospatial dominance and left hemisphere language dominance should be strongly correlated (and perhaps one could be the consequence of the other), in the second the two dominances would be independent. Using functional transcranial Doppler in 75 adults and language and spatial memory tasks, Whitehouse and Bishop conclude in favor of the independence hypothesis. This observation indirectly suggests by itself that manual specialization should be a multidimensional and not unidimensional trait.

Similarly, questions about items' choice or choice between categories (e.g., right/left) versus continuous scores for laterality are common in handedness and laterality of language studies. For instance, the question "which are the best items to assess handedness?" holds also for hemispheric specialization: "which are the best tasks to study language lateralization?" Stroobant, Buijs and Vingerhoets, 2009) report that word generation, sentence generation, reading, and a semantic decision task produce markedly different proportions of left-hemisphere dominance for language, respectively 90%, 80%, 73%, and 67%. Also, for Whitehouse and Bishop, (2009) silent generation of words is recommended in studies of language laterality. It is worth noting that the uni- versus multi-dimensionality problem also appears within language tasks. Concerning the categories versus continuity choice for cerebral specialization, although the amobarbital test and the clinical methods lead to define categories (left, right, and bilateral dominance for language), modern methods of functional exploration of the brain allow to calculate LIs. Low LI's signaling bilateral involvement are associated with an advantage in some studies (e.g., Van Ettinger-Veenstra and al., 2010; Catani and al., 2007), but with a disadvantage in other studies (e.g., Whitehouse and Bishop, 2008); the same holds for subjects with mixed handedness.

It seems reasonable to accept that manual specialization is a more direct manifestation of hemispheric specialization than handedness. For, instance, in children with cerebral palsy, LI at the peg-moving task was strongly correlated with language performance, contrary to manual preference (Dellatolas, Nunes Filho, Souza, Nunes and Willadino Braga, 2005). Also, laterality indexes based on manual skill tasks may be useful in genetic studies, as they give information not included in manual preference. The probability to be left-handed is higher when one of the parents is left-handed. For instance, in a French study, among 1150 children aged 3 to 6 years, the proportion of left-handers was 25% and 20.6% in case of mother's or father's left-handedness respectively, versus 11% and 11.8% when mother or father were right-handed. Among children showing strong right manual preference, the advantage of the right-hand at the peg-moving task was lower when parents were left-handed (Curt, De Agostini, Maccario and Dellatolas, 1995).

III. Gender and Handedness

Many population-based studies of handedness did not report significant difference according to gender. However, a recent meta-analysis of 144 studies concerning a total of more than a million and half subjects, reports more left-handers in males (Papadatou-Patsou, Martin, Munafo and Jones, 2008). We observed this tendency in French children (De Agostini, Paré, Goudot and Dellatolas, 1992), but the opposite tendency (more girls left-handed) in children from India (Singh, Majaury and Dellatolas, 2001). In young adults from France, the degree of right-handedness was stronger in females than in males (Dellatolas, De Agostini, Jallon, Poncet, Rey and Lellouch, 1988). The latter result was congruent with observations based on manual skill tasks in French children, where advantage of the right-hand was stronger in girls than in boys of the same age (De Agostini, Paré, Goudot and Dellatolas, 1992; De Agostini and Dellatolas, 2001). Overall, a slight gender difference on handedness seems to exist, which is not always a difference in the proportion of left-handers.

Is cerebral specialization different in male and female subjects? This question remains open. For instance, a meta-analysis by Sommer, Aleman, Somers, Boks and Kahn (2008) showed no difference between men and women at asymmetry of the Planum temporale, dichotic listening, or functional brain imaging during language tasks. However, Weis, Hausmann, Stoffers, Vohn, Kellermann and Sturm (2008) reported that language lateralization is influenced by estradiol levels during the menstrual cycle in women.

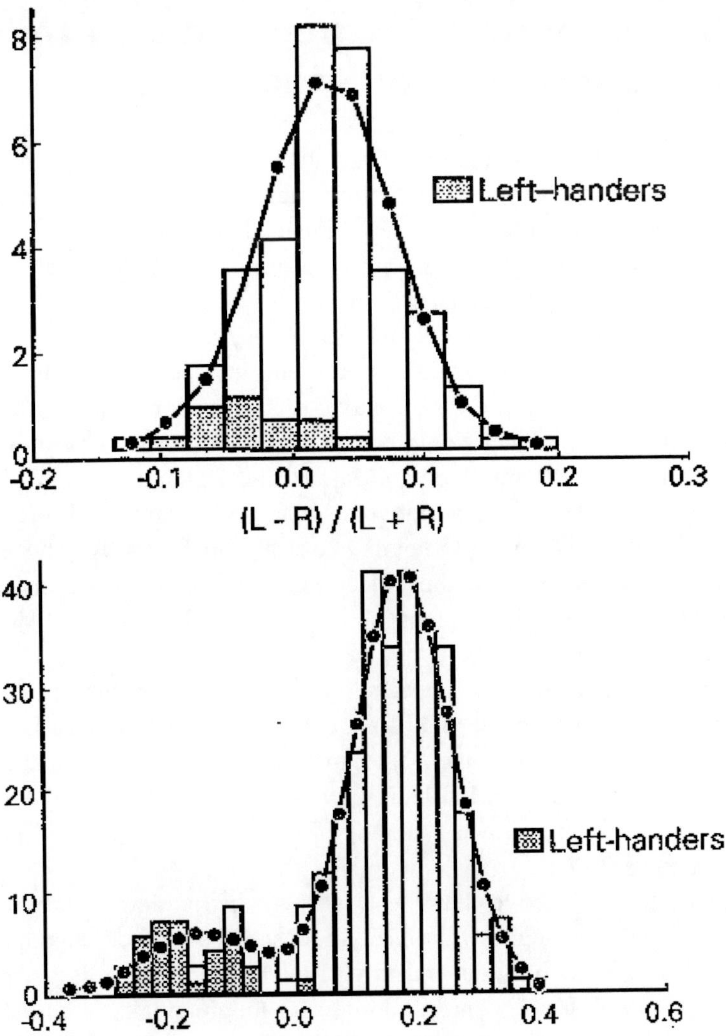

Figure 2. Distribution of the Laterality Index in children aged 4.5 to 5.5 years at the Peg-moving task (N=163) (top) and at a task assessing manual skill using a pencil (N=226) (bottom). At PMT, LI fits with only one normal distribution; at the pencil-task, LI fits better with two normal distributions corresponding to left- and right-handers (from Curt, Maccario and Dellatolas, 1992).

IV. Developmental Aspects in Handedness and Cerebral Specialization

Right-handedness was reported in nonhuman primates for fine manipulation of objects (MacNeilage and al., 1987), for gestures requiring precision (Fagot and Vauclair, 1991; Morange, 1994) or bimanual coordination (Hopkins and Rabinowitz, 1997), and for communication gestures (Meguerditchian and al., 2010; Meguerditchian and Vauclair, 2006).

Manual specialization can be demonstrated very early in infants. For instance, at 4 months, when prehension is not yet present, it is possible to show that left-arm movements towards an object have a localization role, but right-hand movements towards an object would be considered as pre-prehension movements (Morange and Bloch, 1996; Morange-Majoux and Dellatolas, 2010). Kinematic analyzes show that the right-hand movements are more rapid and direct than the left-hand movements (Morange-Majoux, Pezé et Bloch, 2000). At 8 months, a right-hand preference to catch the objects can be shown, which more evident when the baby is engaged in bimanual activities (Fagard, Spelke and Von Hosten, 2009; Fagard and Marks, 2000).

The manual specialization appears not only to the motor but also to the perceptive level: the two-month-old babies memorize haptic information about the shape of an object better with their left hand than with their right hand (Lhote et Stréri, 1998). At 4 months, a left-hand preference to explore rough textures and soft substancies can be shown (Morange-Majoux, Cougnot et Bloch, 1997 ; Morange-Majoux, 2010).

It was mentioned above that the U shaped distribution of the handedness score in the population suggests by itself some snowball effect: degree of manual preference might be activity-dependent and might increase with age in children and in adults as well. Using demonstration tasks longitudinally in children aged 3 to 6 years, it can be shown that although the degree of manual preference increases with age (i.e. the proportion of strong right-handers is higher at 6 years than at 3 years of age), the overall direction of handedness remains relatively constant (i.e. a left-hander at 3 years will remain left-hander at 6 years when a majority criterion is adopted) (Figure 3) (Curt, Maccario and Dellatolas, 1992).

In all our investigations with handedness questionnaires in adults, an age effect on the degree of right-handedness was observed: the proportion of strong right-handers increased with age (Dellatolas, Tubert, Castrenasa, Mesbah, Giallonardo, Lazaratou and Lellouch, 1991). This could mean that the representation of the use of the right hand is stronger in the older than in the younger, and not necessarily that the advantage of the right-hand becomes stronger with age. Such results reflecting handedness activity-dependence and plasticity are important to consider given that it could be erroneously interpreted as a reduction of duration of life in non-strong right-handers (Halpern and Coren, 1998). Is there an age effect on LIs reflecting manual specialization? The answer might be "yes" or "no" according to the specific task used. For instance, in children aged 3 to 6 years, LI increased with age at a task assessing manual skill using a pencil, but not at the peg-moving task (Curt, Maccario and Dellatolas, 1995). Concerning cerebral specialization, strengthening of laterality of verbal and visuospatial functions during childhood and adolescence was reported (Everts, Lidzba, Wilke, Kiefer, Mordasini, Schroth, Perrig and Steinlin, 2009).

V. Pathology Related Issues

Most studies comparing cognitive and academic performances between right- and left-handed children did not report significant differences. However, when manual skill tasks are used and laterality indexes (LI) are calculated, correlations of these LIs with some cognitive tasks are more likely to be observed. For instance, right-hand advantage at the Peg-moving task in French children correlated positively with phonological and visual memory tasks but negatively with vocabulary tasks (De Agostini and Dellatolas, 2001).

Pathological left-handedness may be defined as a change of direction of handedness from right to left as a consequence of a handicap or a neurological disease. It is clear that some handicaps (e.g., absence of the right-hand) or neurological diseases (e.g., cerebral palsy with right hemiplegia, dysfunction of the right-hand due to a left-cerebral hemisphere disease or to a right cerebellar hemisphere disease, etc.) lead to left-handedness in subjects who would probably be right-handed without this handicap or disease. However, this does not suggest that all left-handers have some cerebral dysfunction (Dellatolas, Luciani, Castresana, Rémy, Jallon, Laplane ans Bancaud, 1993). Geschwind and Galaburda (1985) suggested that left-handedness is a risk factor for some auto-immune disorders (e.g., diabetus, Lupus, myasthenia gravis, etc.) or for the occurrence of allergies. However, investigations in the general population and case-control studies did not confirm this (Dellatolas, Annesi, Jallon, Chavance and Lellouch, 1990; Chavance, Dellatolas, Bousser, Amor, Grardel, Kahan, Kahn, Le Floch and Tchobroutsky, 1990; Chavance, Dellatolas and Lellouch, 1992). It was also proposed that left-handers have more accidents, as they live in environment more adapted for the right-handed. In a large population-based study of young adults, we showed that when the consequence of an accident in childhood is the temporary exclusion of the use of the right hand, this may have long lasting consequences on the degree of right-handedness and in some cases may lead to a change of the overall direction of handedness (Dellatolas, Moreau, Jallon and Lellouch, 1993).

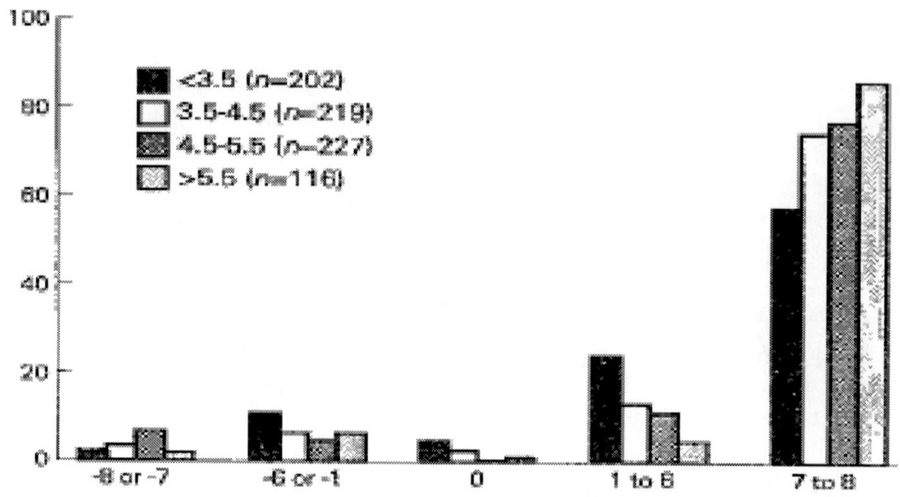

Figure 3. Distribution of the handedness score based on a demonstration task using 8 items (coded –1, 0, 1 for left hand, two hands, and right hand respectively) by age group in children aged 3 to 6 years. The figure shows an increase in the proportion of strong right-handers with age (De Agostini, Paré, Goudot and Dellatolas, 1992).

Similarly, early occurring cerebral lesions can change innate cerebral specialization (e.g., Tracy and al., 2009 ; Möddel, Lineweaver, Schuele, Reinholz and Loddenkemper, 2009), and atypical language lateralization might be related to language or behavioral difficulties. For instance, Whitehouse and Bishop (2008) report that the majority of children with specific language impairment present bilateral or right language dominance.

Conclusion

There is a strong link between manual gestures and language. Handedness, defined as manual preference, is mainly a unidimensional trait, and an example of interaction of genetic, environmental, pathological and activity-related factors determining a human behavior. Manual specialization, evidenced by manual skill tasks, is probably a multidimensional concept more directly linked to hemispheric specialization. Issues related to definition and assessment can partly explain contradictory findings on handedness associations or on the link between handedness and cerebral dominance for language. Furthermore, the role of plasticity and activity-dependence remain debatable. Questions concerning gender differences, developmental aspects, or pathology related issues are similar for handedness and cerebral specialization.

References

Annett, M., (2002). *Handedness and Brain Asymmetry. The right shift Theory*. New York, Taylor and Francis.

Auer, T., Pinter, S., Kovacs, N., Kalmar, Z., Nagy, F., Horvath, R.A., Koszo, B., Kotek, G., Perlaki, G., Koves, M., Kalman, B., Komoly, S., Schwarcz, A., Woermann, F.G. and Janszky, J. (2009) Does obstetric brachial plexus injury influence speech dominance? *Ann Neurol*., 65, 57-66.

Bakan, P. (1990) NonRight-handedness and the continuum of reproductive causality. In S. Coren, A. Searlemann (Eds.). *Left-handedness, behavioral implications and anomalies.* Advances in Psychology, 67, North-Holland, Elsevier.

Broca, P. (1861). Remarques sur le siège du langage articulé, suivie d'une observation d'aphémie (perte de la parole). *Bulletin de la Société Anatomique, 6,* 330-357.

Broca, P. (1865). Sur le siège de la faculté de langage articulé. *Bulletin de la Société d'Anthropologie de Paris, 6,* 377-393.

Buzzard, T. (1882). *Clinical lectures on diseases of the nervous system*. London, Churchill.

Campbell, R., MacSweeney, M. and Waters, D. (2008). Sign language and the brain: a review. *J Deaf Stud Deaf Educ. 13,* 3-20.

Catani, M., Allin M.P., Husain M., Pugliese L., Mesulam M.M., Murray R.M., and Jones D.K. (2007) Symmetries in human brain language pathways correlate with verbal recall. *Proc Natl Acad Sci U S A., 104*, 17163-8.

Chavance, M., Dellatolas, G., Bousser, M.G., Amor, B., Grardel, B., Kahan, A., Kahn, M.F., Le Floch, J.P., and Tchobroutsky, G. (1990) Handedness, immune disorders and information bias. *Neuropsychologia, 28*, 429-441.

Chavance, M., Dellatolas, G., and Lellouch, J. (1992). Correlated non differential misclassifications of disease and exposure: application to a cross-sectional study of the relation between handedness and immune disorders. *International Journal of Epidemiology*, *21*, 537-546.

Comte, J.A. (1828). Recherches anatomo-physiologiques relatives à la prédominance du bras droit sur le bras gauche. *Journal de Physiologie Expérimentale et Pathologie, 8,* 41-80.

Corballis, M.C., (2002). From hand to mouth: The origins of language. Princeton, NJ: Princeton University Press.

Corballis, M..C. (2009). The evolution of language. *Ann.N.Y.Acad.Sci.*, *1156*, 19-43.

Corballis, M.C. (1998). Cerebral asymmetry: Motoring on. *Trends in Cognitive Sciences*, *2*, 1–6.

Coren, S., and Searlemann, A. (1990). *Left-handedness, behavioral implications and anomalies*. Advances in Psychology, 67, North-Holland, Elsevier.

Crosson, B. (2008). An intention manipulation to change lateralization of word production in nonfluent aphasia: current status. *Semin Speech Lang,. 3,* 188-200.

Curt, F., De Agostini, M., Maccario, J., and Dellatolas, G. (1995). Parental hand preference and manual functional asymmetry in preschool children. *Behavior Genetics, 25,* 525-536.

Curt, F., Maccario, J., and Dellatolas, G. (1992). Distributions of hand preference and hand skill asymmetry in preschool children : theoretical implications. *Neuropsychologia, 30*, 27-34.

Curt, F., Mesbah, M., Lellouch, L., and Dellatolas, G. (1997). Handedness Scale: how many and which items. *Laterality, 2,* 137-154.

De Agostini M., and Dellatolas G. (2001). Lateralities in normal children and their role on cognitive performance. *Developmental Neuropsychology, 20*, 429-444.

De Agostini, M., Hassan Khamis, A., Ahui, A.M., and Dellatolas, G. (1997). Environmental influences in hand preference: an African point of view. *Brain and Cognition, 35*, 151-167.

De Agostini, M., Paré, C., Goudot, D., and Dellatolas, G. (1992). Manual preference and skill development in preschool children. *Developmental Neuropsychology, 8,* 41-57.

Dehaene-Lambertz, G., Dehaene, S., and Hertz-Pannier, L. (2002). Functional neuroimaging of speech perception in infants. *Science, 298*, 2013-5.

Dellatolas, G., Luciani, S., Castresana, A., Rémy, C., Jallon, P., Laplane, D., and Bancaud, J. (1993). Pathological left-handedness: left-handedness correlatives in adult epileptics. *Brain, 116*, 1565-1574.

Dellatolas, G., Annesi, I., Jallon, P., Chavance, M., and Lellouch, J. (1990). An epidemiological reconsideration of the Geschwind-Galaburda theory of cerebral lateralization. *Archives of Neurology, 47*, 778-782.

Dellatolas, G., De Agostini, M., Curt, F., Kremin, H., Letierce, A., Maccario, J., and Lellouch, J. (2003). Manual skill, hand skill asymmetry, and cognitive performances in young children. *Laterality, 8,* 317-338.

Dellatolas, G., De Agostini, M., Jallon, P., Poncet, M., Rey, M., and Lellouch, J (1988). Mesure de la préférence manuelle par autoquestionnaire dans la population française adulte. *Revue de Psychologie Appliquée, 38*, 117-136.

Dellatolas, G., and Lazaratou, H. (1989). Mesure et fréquence de la préférence manuelle gauche en Grèce. *Iatriki, 56*, 257-264.

Dellatolas, G., Moreau, T., Jallon, P., and Lellouch, J. (1993). Upper limb injuries and handedness plasticity. *British Journal of Psychology, 84*, 201-205.

Dellatolas, G., Nunes Filho, G., Souza, L., Nunes, LG., and Willadino Braga, L. (2005). Manual skill, hand skill asymmetry, and neuropsychological testing in school-children with spastic cerebral palsy. *Laterality, 2005*, 10: 161-82.

Dellatolas, G., Tubert, P., Castresana, A., Mesbah, M., Giallonardo, T., Lazaratou, H., and Lellouch J. (1991). Age and cohort effects in adult handedness. *Neuropsychologia,* 29, 255-261.

Dellatolas, G., Tubert-Bitter, P., Curt, F., and De Agostini, M. (1997). Evolution and degree of hand preference in children: Methodological and theoretical issues. *Neuropsychological Rehabilitation,* 7, 387-399.

Dellatolas, G., Vanluchene, J., and Coutin, T. (1996). Visual and motor components in simple line bisection: an investigation in normal adults. *Cognitive Brain Research, 4,* 49-56.

Dubois J., Hertz-Pannier, L., Cachia, A., Mangin, J.F., Le Bihan, D., and Dehaene-Lambertz, G. (2009). Structural asymmetries in the infant language and sensori-motor networks. *Cerebral Cortex, 19*, 414-23.

Everts, R., Lidzba, K., Wilke, M., Kiefer, C., Mordasini, M., Schroth, G., Perrig, W., and Steinlin, M. (2009). Strengthening of laterality of verbal and visuospatial functions during childhood and adolescence. *Hum Brain Mapp.*, *30*, 473-83.

Fagard, J., and Marks, A. (2000). Unimanual and bimanual tasks and the assessement of handedness in toddlers. *Developmental Science*, *3*: 137-147.

Fagard, J., Spelke, E., andvon Hofsten, C. (2009). Reaching and grasping a moving object in 6-, 8-, and 10- month-old infants: laterality and performance. *Infant Behavior and Development, 32,* 137-146.

Fagot, J., and Vauclair, J. (1991). Manual laterality in nonhuman primates : a distinction between handedness and manual specialization. *Psychological Bulletin, 109*, 76-89.

Gallese, V., Fadiga, L., Fogassi, L., and Rizzolatti, G., (1996). Action recognition in the premotor cortex. *Brain, 119*, 593–609.

Geschwind, N., and Behan, P.O. (1982). Left-handedness: association with immune disease, migraine, and developmental learning disorder. *Proc Natl Acad Sci* USA, 79, 5097-5100.

Geschwind, N., and Levitsky, W. (1968). Human brain: left-right asymmetry in temporal speech region. *Science, 161*, 186-187.

Geschwind, N., and Galaburda, A.M. (1985). Cerebral lateralization: biological mecanisms, associations, and pathology. *Arch Neurol, 42*, 428-459, 521-552, 634-654.

Goldin-Meadow S., Mylander C., and Butcher C. (1995). The resilience of combinatorial structure at the word level: morphology in self-styled gesture systems. *Cognition, 56*, 195-262.

Goldin-Meadow, S., and Mylandre, C. (1998). Spontaneous sign systems created by deaf children in two cultures. *Nature,* 391, 279-281.

Goldin-Meadow, S. (1999). The role of gesture in communication and thinking. *Trends in Cognitive Sciences, 3,* 419-429.

Halpern, D.F., and Coren, S. (1988). Do right-handers live longer ? *Nature, 333*, 213.

Harris, L.J. (1980). Left-handedness: early theories, facts, and fancies. In J. Herron (Ed). *Neuropsychology of left-handedness*. New York, Academic Press.

Hécaen, H., and Ajuriaguerra, J. (1963). *Les gauchers : prévalence manuelle et dominance cérébrale*. Paris, Presses Universitaires de France.

Hécaen, H. (1984). *Les gauchers*. Paris, Presse Universitaires de France.

Iverson, J.M., and Goldin-Meadow S. (1998). Why people gesture when they speak. *Nature*, 396, 228.

Iverson, J.M., and Goldin-Meadow, S. (2005). Gesture paves the way for language development. *Psychological Science*, 16, 367-371.

Jackson, J. (1905). *Ambidexterity or two handedness and two brainedness*. London, Kegan and Co.

Leurat, F., and Gratiolet, P. (1857). *Anatomie comparée du système nerveux, considéré dans ses rapports avec l'intelligence*. Paris, Baillère.

Lhote, M., and Streri, A. (1998). Haptic memory and handedness in 2-month-old infants. *Laterality, 3,* 173-192.

Lust, J.M., Geuze, R.H., Van de Beek, C., Cohen-Kettenis, PT., Groothuis, A.G., and Bouma, A. (2009). Sex specific effect of prenatal testosterone on language lateralization in children. *Neuropsychologia*. 2009, 23.

McNeilage, P.F., Studdert-Kennedy., M.G.., and Lindblom., B. (1987). Primate handedness reconsidered. *Behavioral and Brain Sciences, 10,* 247-303.

Meguerditchian, A., Vauclair, J., and Hopkins, W.D. (2010). Captive chimpanzees use their right hand to communicate with each other: implications for the origin of the cerebral substrate for language. *Cortex, 46,* 40-48.

Meguerditchian, A., and Vauclair, J. (2006). Baboons communicate with their right hand. *Behav Brain Res., 171*, 170-174.

Mercure, E., Ashwin, E., Dick, F., Halit, H., Auyeung, B., Baron-Cohen, S., and Johnson, M.H. (2009). IQ fetal testosterone and individual variability in children's functional lateralization. *Neuropsychologia*, *47,* 2537-43.

Möddel, G., Lineweaver, T., Schuele, S.U., Reinholz, J., and Loddenkemper, T. (2009). Atypical language lateralization in epilepsy patients. *Epilepsia, 50,* 1505-16.

Morange., F. (1994). Handedness in two chimpanzees in captivity. In J.R. Anderson., J.J. Roeder, B. Thierry and N. Herrenschmidt (Eds.), *Current primatology: Behavioral neuroscience physiology and reproduction, Vol. 3.* Strasbourg: Université Louis Pasteur, pp. 61-68.

Morange, F. and Bloch, H. (1996). Lateralization of the approach movement and the prehension movement in infants from 4 to 7 months. *Early Development and Parenting, 5(2)*: 81-92.

Morange-Majoux, F. and Dellatolas, G. (2010). Right-Left approaching and reaching hand movements of 4-month infants in free and constrained conditions. *Brain and Cognition, 72, 419-422.*

Morange-Majoux, F. (2010). Manual exploration of softness and hardness in infants 4 to 6 months of age, *Laterality, 12, 1-21.*

Morange-Majoux, F., Cougnot, P. and Bloch, H. (1997). Hand tactual exploration of textures in infants from 4 to 6 months. *Early Development and Parenting, 6,* 152-161.

Morange-Majoux, F., Pezé, A. and Bloch, H. (2000). Organization of left and right hand movement in a prehension task : A longitudinal study from 20 to 32 weeks. *Laterality*, *4*, 1-12.

Oldfield, R.C. (1971). The assessment and analysis of handedness: the Edinburgh Inventory. *Neuropsychologia, 9*, 97-113.

Papadatou-Pastou, M., Martin, M., Munafò, M.R., and Jones, G.V. (2008). Sex differences in left-handedness: a meta-analysis of 144 studies. *Psychol Bull,. 134*, 677-99.

Previc, F.H. (1991). A general theory concerning the origins of cerebral lateralization in humans. *Psychological Review, 98*, 299-334.

Rasmussen, T., and Milner, B. (1977). The role of early left-brain injury in determining lateralization of cerebral speech functions. *Ann N.Y. Acad. Sci., 199*, 355-369.

Reade, C. (1878). *The coming man*. Letters to the Editor of Harper's Weekly.

Rey, M., Dellatolas, G., Bancaud, J., and Talairach, J. (1988). Hemispheric lateralization of motor and speech functions after early brain lesions : study of 73 epileptic patients with intracarotid amytal test. *Neuropsychologia, 26*, 167-172.

Rowe, M.L., and Goldin-Meadow, S. (2009). Early gesture selectively predicts later language learning. *Developmental Science 12*, 182-187.

Saucier, D., and Elias, L., (2001). Lateral and sex differences in manual gesture during conversation. *Laterality*, *6*, 239-245.

Singh, M., Manjary, M., and Dellatolas, G. (2001). Lateral preferences among indian school children., *Cortex, 37*, 231-41.

Sommer, I.E., Aleman, A., Somers, M., Boks, M.P., and Kahn, R.S. (2008). Sex differences in handedness, asymmetry of the planum temporale and functional language lateralization. *Brain Res., 1206*, 76-88.

Stroobant, N., Buijs, D., and Vingerhoets, G. (2009). Variation in brain lateralization during various language tasks: a functional transcranial Doppler study, *Behav Brain Res., 199*,190-6.

Tracy, J.I., Waldron, B., Glosser, D., Sharan, A., Mintzer, S., Zangaladze, A., Skidmore, C., Siddiqui, I., Caris, E., and Sperling, M.R. (2009). Hemispheric lateralization and language skill coherence in temporal lobe epilepsy. *Cortex, 45*, 1178-89.

Turkewitz, G. (1988). A prenatal source of the development of hemispheric specialization. In D.L. Molfesen S.J. Segalowitz (Eds). *Brain lateralization in children: developmental implications*. New York, Guilford.

van Ettinger-Veenstra HM, Ragnehed M, Hällgren M, Karlsson T, Landtblom AM,

Lundberg P, Engström M. (2010). Right-hemispheric brain activation correlates to language performance. *Neuroimage*, 3481-3418.

Wada, J., and Rasmussen, T. (1960). Intracarotid injection of sodium amytal for the lateralization of cerebral speech dominance. *J Neurosurg.*, *17*, 242-282.

Warrier, C., Wong, P., Penhune, V., Zatorre, R., Parrish, T., Abrams, D., and Kraus, N. (2009) Relating structure to function: Heschl's gyrus and acoustic processing. *J Neurosci.*, *29*, 61-9.

Weis, S., Hausmann, M., Stoffers, B., Vohn, R., Kellermann, T., and Sturm, W. (2008). Estradiol modulates functional brain organization during the menstrual cycle: an analysis of interhemispheric inhibition. *J Neurosci.*, *28*, 13401-10.

Whitehouse, AJ., and Bishop, D.V. (2008). Cerebral dominance for language function in adults with specific language impairment or autism. *Brain, 131*, 3193-200.

Whitehouse, A.J., and Bishop, D.V. (2009). Hemispheric division of function is the result of independent probabilistic biases. *Neuropsychologia, 47*, 1938-1943.

In: Handedness: Theories, Genetics and Psychology ISBN: 978-1-61470-502-4
Editors: J. Dunham and T. Davenport

Chapter IV

Handedness and Mental Rotation

***Nobuaki Shimoda*[1], *Kotaro Takeda*[2] *and Hiroyuki Kato*[3]**
[1]Department of Occupational Therapy, Kyorin University, Japan
[2]Department of Motor Control and Rehabilitation, ATR Computational Neuroscience Laboratories, Japan
[3]Department of Neurology, International University of Health and Welfare Hospital, Japan

Abstract

Right-handed and left-handed individuals have been found to differ in their ability to perform tasks with the dominant and non-dominant hand. Laterality of brain function in verbal tasks and spatial cognitive tasks also appears to differ according to handedness. Spatial cognitive tasks involving mental rotation of shapes have been used to study the relationships of handedness, handedness of immediate family and sex to reaction time and correct response rate. Cerebral activation during these tasks has also been studied. The relationship between handedness and reaction time has also been investigated in tasks involving mental rotation of hand images, where the subject is presented with a photograph or drawing of a hand rotated at a specific angle and must judge whether it is a left or right hand. We have previously published studies on brain activation during the mental rotation of shapes and on reaction times in the mental rotation of hand pictures in left- and right-handed subjects. In this paper we review the literature relating to the relationship of handedness to reaction times and brain activation in mental rotation tasks.

Introduction

Motor competence in the dominant and non-dominant hand differs between left- and right-handed individuals. Lateralization of brain function in verbal tasks and spatial cognitive tasks also differs according to handedness. Right-handers show a large difference in motor competence between the dominant and non-dominant hand, but left-handers do not exhibit such large differences in competence or in frequency of use of the dominant and non-dominant hand [23,24,38]. In regard to lateralization of brain function, there is evidence that right-handers are left-hemisphere dominant in verbal tasks [4] and right-hemisphere dominant in spatial cognitive tasks [25]. Some studies suggest that hemispheric dominance in left-handers differs from that of right-handers in verbal tasks [3,67], while studies on spatial cognitive tasks are equivocal, some finding no clearly dominant hemisphere in left-handers when compared to right-handers [27], and others finding no difference between left- and right-handers [62,75].

One spatial cognitive task involves mental rotation of a three-dimensional object [63] in which a pair of objects are presented at different angles of rotation and the subject is required to determine whether the two are identical or mirror images. This task has been used in studies on the relationships of handedness, handedness of immediate family and sex to reaction time and correct response rates [7,8,9,10,11,55], and in research on brain activation during task performance [6,12,14,26].

Another mental rotation task uses hand pictures; the subject is presented with a series of photographs or drawings depicting hands at various angles of rotation and is required to determine whether the hand is a left or right hand. Measurements of reaction time and brain function during these tasks have indicated that subjects may be simulating the action of superimposing their own hand on the physical image during hand mental rotation [15,16,30,31,51,59]. It is possible that handedness has a greater influence on tasks using hand images than on those requiring object rotation. While this is an intriguing possibility, previous hand mental rotation studies have primarily used right-handed subjects.

In measuring the brain activity of left- and right-handers during mental rotation of objects, we found that left-handers showed slight left-hemisphere dominance in the frontal and parietal lobes, whereas right-handers showed dominant activation in the right hemisphere in both the frontal and parietal lobes

[64]. In regard to reaction times in hand mental rotation tasks, we have also reported that right-handers reacted more quickly to photographs of the right hand than to photographs of the left hand, whereas left-handers did not show this difference. In addition, both left- and right-handers appear to be simulating rotation of their own hands when performing these tasks [69]. In the present paper we review the relationship of handedness to reaction time and brain activity in mental rotation tasks [81].

Mental Rotation Task of Three-dimensional Objects

Mental rotation tasks using three-dimensional objects, first described by Shepard and Metzler [63], require the subject to decide whether items in a pair of three-dimensional objects are the same or different, and the decision response time is measured. The two objects are identical or mirror images, and are presented at mutually different angles of rotation. Reaction times were found to be proportional to the angle of rotation between the two images, which raised the possibility that subjects were performing the task by mentally rotating one object to superimpose it on the other. After this pioneering study, a number of follow-up studies using the same measurement paradigm support Shepard and Metzler's findings that reaction times increased with the angle of rotation [13,18,29,35,59]. As well as three-dimensional objects, other stimuli have been used, such as alphabet letters [13], abstract line drawings [29], and drawings of hands [59].

Results conflict as to whether right-handers and left-handers differ in their ability to perform mental rotation of objects. In a study with 12 right-handers and 12 left-handers, Herrmann and van Dyke measured reaction times in a mental rotation task using abstract line drawings and found that left-handers reacted more quickly than right-handers [29]. However, in a study measuring reaction times involving a mental rotation of line drawings with right-handers, familial left-handers, and non-familial left-handers, Jones and Anuza found that right-handers had faster reaction times than the other two groups [35]. In an investigation of the association between ambidextrous tendencies and scores on object mental rotation task, McGee found that subjects with strong ambidextrous tendencies had good scores [45].

Sex differences in object mental rotation tasks have also been studied, with much evidence accumulated that males perform better than females [54,76,77]. Some research on the effect of handedness on object mental rotation ability suggests that differences depend on whether the subject is male or female. For example, Sanders and colleagues reported that male left-handers had better test scores than male right-handers, whereas among females, right-handers scored better than left-handers [57]. Lewis and Harris investigated performance in object mental rotation among 56 of the highest scoring university students (top 7%) in the US SAT tests: in males, right-handers had a higher correct response rate than left-handers, whereas in females the left-handers scored more highly [41]. In males, pure left-handers have been found to have lower mental rotation scores than left-handers with ambidextrous tendencies and right-handers, but these differences were not apparent in females [65]. A comparison of subjects undergoing sex hormone therapy for male-to-female sex reassignment and a control group of male subjects found no intergroup differences in ability to perform mental rotation of objects [79].

In an attempt to explain sex differences and individual differences in spatial cognitive ability, Casey and colleagues conducted a series of studies [7,8,9,10,11,55] building on the theories of Annet [1,2], who posits the existence of allelic genes for handedness, and Sherman [61], who attributes individual differences in female spatial cognitive ability to environmental factors. These studies shared the hypothesis that in the case of females, right-handers with non-right-handed immediate family would have spatial cognitive ability superior to right-handers and non-right-handers whose immediate family were all right-handers, and that this superior ability would be limited to subjects who had had a good deal of experience of activities requiring spatial cognitive ability (e.g. majoring in mathematics or frequently engaging in play or leisure activities requiring spatial cognitive ability).

A study of university students majoring or not majoring in mathematics found that mathematics majors who were female, right-handed, and with non-right-handed immediate family performed better in object mental rotation tasks than female right-handers with only right-handed immediate family and female non-right-handers; among non-mathematics majors there were no differences between the three groups; and males showed no differences between the three groups, whether mathematics majors or not. [7]. Similarly, in a study of female high-school students taking the preparatory program for a mathematics course, right-handers with non-right-handed immediate family performed better in object mental rotation tasks than right-handers with only right-handed immediate family and non-right-handers [9].

When female university students were divided into a high-experience group and low-experience group based on self-assessment of experience in activities using spatial cognition (e.g. carpentry), in the high-experience group right-handers with non-right-handed immediate family performed better in object mental rotation than right-handers with only right-handed immediate family, but no such difference was seen in the low-experience group [8]. Furthermore, subjects with non-right-handed immediate family who reported that they had engaged in spatial cognitive activities with their siblings performed better in object mental rotation than subjects with non-right-handed immediate family who reported that they had not engaged in spatial cognitive activities with their siblings and subjects with only right-handed immediate family [11].

To understand how right-handed females with only right-handed immediate family differed from right-handed females with non-right-handed immediate family in terms of the strategies used for object mental rotation tasks, Pezaris and Casey investigated performance differences when subjects who were doing object mental rotations were given simultaneous verbal interference trials or simultaneous spatial interference trials [55]. The results showed that right-handed females with high mathematics or science achievement and with non-right-handed immediate family performed more poorly in spatial interference trials than in verbal interference trials, whereas right-handed females with high mathematics or science achievement and with only right-handed immediate family showed the opposite: better performance in spatial interference trials than in verbal interference trials. The right-handed females with low mathematics or science achievement also performed more poorly in verbal interference trials than in spatial interference trials. These results suggest that right-handed females with non-right-handed immediate family relied more on spatial cognitive ability to perform these tasks, while right-handed females with only right-handed immediate family and right handed females with low math or science achievement relied more on language function. On the other hand, Li and colleagues suggested that handedness of immediate family had no influence on test scores in mental rotation tasks [42].

Cerebral Activation during Mental Rotation Tasks of Three-dimensional Objects

Since the 1990s, a number of studies have used functional brain imagine techniques such as positron emission tomography (PET) and functional magnetic resonance imaging (fMRI) in the measurement of cerebral activation during mental rotation tasks, with particular attention given to activity in the parietal association area [6,12,14,26]. Cohen and colleagues reported activity in the superior parietal lobule in all 8 subjects when measuring brain activity during object mental rotation tasks with fMRI [12], and Carpenter and colleagues found that superior parietal lobule activity was influenced by the amount of mental rotation [6]. Other studies have described activity in the primary sensorimotor area, premotor area, occipital lobe, and parietal lobe [32,80].

Studies of right-handed subjects repeatedly show that brain activity is dominant in the right hemisphere in tasks using shapes and objects [17,64], and letters and numbers [26]. However, some researchers doubt there is pure right-hemisphere dominance, since these results are affected by factors such as the poor temporal resolution of PET and fMRI [32], while others suggest that the contribution of each hemisphere is dependent on the angle of rotation [19].

Hécaen and colleagues examined hemispheric dominance of spatial cognitive function in left-handers by comparing spatial cognitive dysfunction in left-handers and right-handers with unilateral brain damage [27]. They found that most right-handers had impairment of spatial cognitive function due to right-brain damage, whereas left-handers with similar impairment were about equally divided between right-brain and left-brain damage, perhaps indicating that hemispheric dominance of spatial cognitive function is not so clear cut in left-handers as it is in right-handers. However, research on event-related potentials in figure-matching tasks [75] and spatial cognitive tests using a tachistoscope for momentary stimulus presentation [62] found no hemispheric differences between left- and right-handers. Overall, there is a paucity of research on brain activity in left-handers during mental rotation of objects.

Studies of sex differences in brain function during mental rotation tasks have revealed that males and females exhibit similar brain function during task performance, but sex differences have been reported in brain function in areas such as the superior and inferior parietal lobes including intraparietal sulcus, inferior frontal gyrus, inferior parietal gyrus, and primary motor area, and it is suggested that these differences could arise from anatomical differences and differences in task performance strategies [36,71,78]. Johnson and colleagues used event-related potential to examine the sex differences of brain activity during mental rotation tasks involving alphabetic characters [34]. They found that in both right-handed and left-handed females, the left hemisphere was dominant when participants were asked to press a button for task execution using their dominant hand, and the right hemisphere was dominant when using the non-dominant hand, whereas both right- and left-handed males showed right hemisphere dominance irrespective of which hand was used for pressing the button. Although these results are interpreted as indicating male-female differences in the laterality of motor control in the dominant and non-dominant hand, differences between left-handers are right-handers are not mentioned.

We have used near-infrared spectroscopy (NIRS) to compare differences in brain activity between left- and right-handers when performing mental rotation of objects [64]. NIRS allows measurement of changes in blood concentrations of oxygenated hemoglobin (Δ[Oxy-Hb]) and deoxygenated hemoglobin in response to neural activity by scanning the cerebral cortex with near-infrared light [43]. The subjects were presented with 4 objects (one was in the upper panel and the other three objects were in the lower panel), and asked to determine if the top object was identical to any of the three below (the objects were based on those used by Vandenburg and Kuse [74]). NIRS measurement was set up to cover the following regions of interest (ROI): the primary motor area, premotor area, frontal lobe including frontal association area, primary somatosensory area, superior parietal lobule, angular gyrus, and parietal lobe including supramarginal gyrus. A right hemisphere laterality index (RI) was defined as RI = (NR-NL) / (NR+NL) (a modification of the Laterality Index [68]) using the number of Δ[Oxy-Hb] measurement channels that showed significant activation during the task. Here, NR and NL are the number of channels showing significant changes in the right and left hemispheres, respectively. The index ranged from -1 to 1, with positive values indicating right hemisphere dominance and negative values indicating left hemisphere dominance. The RI (mean ± SD) in right-handers indicated right-hemisphere dominance in the frontal lobe (RI = 0.31 ± 0.25) and parietal lobe (RI = 0.28 ± 0.37), while left-handers showed slight left-hemisphere dominance in the frontal lobe (RI = -0.12 ± 0.18) and parietal lobe (RI = -0.22 ± 0.22). The RIs of right-handers in the frontal and parietal lobes were significantly larger than those of left-handers. These results suggest that hemispheric laterality in mental rotation tasks differs according to handedness.

Mental Rotation Task of Hand Pictures

In mental rotation tasks of hand pictures, the subject is presented with a photograph or drawing of a hand at a given angle of rotation and is asked to determine whether it is a left or right hand. Unlike the results for object mental rotation tasks, reaction times in the hand tasks became slower when the angle of rotation could not be easily copied by the subject moving their actual hand [15,16,52,59]. Reaction times were also dependent on the subject's arm posture during the task [15,16,30,31]. These results raised the possibility that subjects were simulating the action of superimposing their own hand on the photograph or drawing during mental rotation. Correct response rates and reaction times have also been measured in subjects with central motor disorders such as stroke [56,72], Parkinson's disease [28], and cerebral palsy [47,66], as well as in upper limb amputees [48] and subjects with congenitally absent hands [20]. Scores were low in patients with central motor disorders compared to healthy subjects [56, 66], and in subjects with left-brain damage compared to those with right-brain damage [72], while dominant-hand amputees had slower reaction times than non-dominant-hand amputees [48] and were slower to react when the hand image presented was on the same side as the absent hand [20].

Gentilucci and colleagues hypothesized that, since right-handers show large differences in motor skills between the left and right hands whereas left-handers show comparatively less difference, these differences would also manifest in reaction times during mental rotation of a hand holding an implement [22]. To test this, they measured the time taken to decide if a hand photographed holding an implement such as a table tennis bat was a left or right hand, using 10 right-handers and 10 left-handers as subjects. The hand photographs were prepared so that the hand shape either conformed (congruent condition) or did not conform (incongruent condition) to the implement being held. The congruent condition was, for example, a photograph of a hand correctly gripping a table tennis bat, whereas the incongruent condition showed the bat held between thumb and index finger. These congruent and incongruent photographs were also divided into those depicting a functionally natural or unnatural position. For example, a functionally natural position was depicted by a photograph of a hand gripping the bat away from the hitting surface in the usual way, whereas a functionally unnatural position was depicted by a bat reversed 180 degrees so that the hitting surface was held. It was found that right-handers reacted more quickly to right-hand photographs than to left-hand photographs, but no such difference was seen in left-handers. In congruent right-hand photographs, right-handers also reacted more quickly to functionally natural positions than functionally unnatural positions. In contrast, left-handers showed no difference in reaction times to functionally natural and functionally unnatural positions in congruent left-hand photographs. Based on these results, the authors speculate that right-handers could be performing these tasks while visualizing the movement of their dominant right hand, whereas left-handers are perhaps using a more visual analysis.

In a study of 10 left-handers and 16 right-handers, Ionta and Blanke measured reaction times in a left-right decision task using photographs of hands and feet while having subjects alter their hand postures [31]. Two hand posture conditions were compared: right hand behind back with left hand resting on lap, and left hand behind back with right hand resting on lap. In agreement with Gentilucci and colleagues' results [22], the study found that right-handers reacted more quickly to photographs of the right hand than those of the left hand, and left-handers showed no such difference. Right-handers also reacted more slowly to photographs of the right hand when the subject's right hand was behind the back than on the lap, but this effect was not seen with foot photographs. Left-handers showed no difference in reaction times to photographs of the left hand irrespective of whether the subject's left hand was behind the back or on the lap, and no difference with the foot photographs. The authors speculate that these results could arise from differences in frequency of use of the dominant hand among right-handers and left-handers.

We compared reaction times in mental hand rotation tasks performed by 16 right-handers and 15 left-handers [64] identified as such using the Edinburgh Inventory [49]. The stimuli presented were 512 hand photographs consisting of combinations of four factors: 1) right or left hand, 2) palm or back of hand, 3) fingers extended or flexed, 4) orientation (upright, 0°; CW, 90°; CCW, -90°; inverted, 180°). Subjects were asked to determine if each photograph was a left or right hand, and their reaction times were measured. It was found that right-handers had significantly slower reaction times to photographs of the left hand than to those of the right hand, but no such difference was seen in left-handers. Mental and actual hand movement speeds are also thought to correlate strongly [52]. For example, in right-handers the speed of visualized movement is slower in the left hand than the right hand, just as it is in physical movement tasks [44]. Furthermore, right-handers show a large difference in motor skills between the dominant (right) hand and non-dominant (left) hand, implying strong lateralization to the dominant hand side, whereas left-handers do not show such a large difference between the dominant hand and non-dominant hand [23,24,38]. These findings suggest that our results—that reaction times differ between left-handers and right-handers—arise from differences in the lateralization of manual motor skills. We also found that both right-handers and left-handers reacted more quickly to photographs of the right hand in the CCW position than in the CW position, but more quickly to photographs of the left hand in the CW position than in the CCW position. These results suggest that both left-handers and right-handers perform these tasks by imagining the rotation of their own hand, that is, by using a motor imagery.

Cerebral Activation during Mental Rotation Tasks of Hand Pictures

Measurement of brain function during mental rotation of hand pictures has revealed cerebral activation in the parietal lobes and premotor area as is seen in motor imagery tasks [5,16,37,40,53], and together with reaction times, these findings support the notion that subjects perform these tasks by simulating the act of superimposing their own hand on the hand image presented.

There is much evidence that brain function in the parietal lobes and premotor area is left-hemisphere dominant in right-handers [5,16,40]. Using fMRI to measure brain activity during mental rotation of line drawings of hands, de Lange and colleagues detected brain activation bilaterally in the dorsal premotor areas and parietal sulci [16]. However, in the right hemisphere these structures showed weaker activation in response to drawings of the right hand than to drawings of the left hand, whereas in the left hemisphere they were strongly activated in response to both sets of drawings. This paper also reports that activity in the left parietal sulcus significantly increased when subjects changed arm posture during tasks. When comparing brain function by PET measurement in a baseline task in which subjects judged whether two non-rotated line drawings of hands were identical or different, and an experimental task where the two drawings were separated by an angle of rotation, Kosslyn and colleagues reported a significant increase in blood flow in the left premotor area and left parietal lobe [40]. Bonda and colleagues also found that increased blood flow increase was predominant in the left parietal lobe rather than in the right parietal lobe during task performance [5]. Research on brain-damaged subjects has also found that subjects with left-brain damage produce fewer correct responses than those with right-brain damage in hand mental rotation tasks [72], and also exhibit different reaction time patterns to normal subjects [47, 66], providing further evidence that the left hemisphere is dominant in these tasks. However, another study found no hemispheric dominance [70].

Brain activity in the primary motor cortex has also been studied during mental rotation of hand images. Tomasino and colleagues found that transcranial magnetic stimulation (TMS) to the primary motor area in the left hemisphere slowed reaction times in hand mental rotation tasks but had no effect on mental rotation of letters, whereas TMS to the right primary motor area had no effect on either hand or letter rotation [73]. Ganis and colleagues reported that TMS applied to the left primary motor area influenced reaction times in hand mental rotation, but not in foot mental rotation [21]. Kosslyn and colleagues found that brain activity in the left precentral gyrus was greater in mental rotation of hand images than of objects [40]. These results suggest that the left primary motor area contributes to performance of hand mental rotation tasks. However, some of the literature reports no activity in the primary motor area [53], or considers that brain activity in the primary motor area is associated with the actual movement of button-pressing during tasks [15], or finds that TMS in the left primary motor area does not alter reaction times [58].

Most of this research is on right-handed individuals, and though brain function has been measured during hand mental rotation in both left- and right-handers [60], the study investigated the effects of task pacing on brain function and did not discuss functional differences between left- and right-handers.

Clinical Applicability of Mental Rotation Tasks

Motor imagery has been used as one of the recent therapeutic approaches for upper limb hemiparesis building on knowledge gained from advances in the measurement of brain function. The neural substrates of motor imagery are thought to be the same as in motor preparation for actual movement [33], and application of this knowledge to the treatment of upper limb dysfunction in hemiparetic patients is beginning to bear fruit [39, 50]. The literature reviewed in this paper strongly suggests that subjects performing mental rotation of hand images simulate the movement of their own hands, and demonstrates that motor related brain areas are activated during these tasks. Utilizing this knowledge, hand mental rotation tasks have been used to try to alleviate pain due to complex regional pain syndrome type 1 [46]; this method may also be applicable to treatment of upper limb dysfunction in hemiparetic patients. However, application of this method to the treatment of hemiparesis will require more knowledge of cerebral activation during task performance, and we await future research in this area.

References

[1] Annett, M. (1985). *Left, right, hand, and brain: The right shift theory.* London: Erlbaum.

[2] Annett, M. (1994). Handedness as a continuous variable with dextral shift: sex, generation, and family handedness in subgroups of left- and right-handers. *Behav Genet, 24*, 51-63.

[3] Basic, S., Hajnsek, S., Poljakovic, Z., Basic, M., Culic, V., and Zadro, I. (2004). Determination of cortical language dominance using functional transcranial Doppler sonography in left-handers. *Clin Neurophysiol, 115*, 154-160.

[4] Bethmann, A., Tempelmann, C., De Bleser, R., Scheich, H., and Brechmann, A. (2007). Determining language laterality by fMRI and dichotic listening. *Brain Res, 1133*, 145-157.

[5] Bonda, E., Petrides, M., Frey, S., and Evans, A. (1995). Neural correlates of mental transformations of the body-in-space. *Proc Natl Acad Sci U S A, 92*, 11180-11184.

[6] Carpenter, P.A., Just, M. A., Keller, T. A., Eddy, W., and Thulborn, K. (1999). Graded functional activation in the visuospatial system with the amount of task demand. *J Cogn Neurosci, 11*, 9-24.

[7] Casey, M.B., and Brabeck, M.M. (1989). Exceptions to the male advantage on a spatial task: family handedness and college major as factors identifying women who excel. *Neuropsychologia, 27*, 689-696.

[8] Casey, M.B., and Brabeck, M.M. (1990). Women who excel on a spatial task: proposed genetic and environmental factors. *Brain Cogn, 12*, 73-84.

[9] Casey, M.B., Colon, D., and Goris, Y. (1992). Family handedness as a predictor of mental rotation ability among minority girls in a math-science training program. *Brain Cogn, 18*, 88-96.

[10] Casey, M.B., Pezaris, E., and Nuttall, R.L. (1992). Spatial ability as a predictor of math achievement: the importance of sex and handedness patterns. *Neuropsychologia, 30*, 35-45.

[11] Casey, M.B., Nuttall, R.L., and Pezaris E. (1999). Evidence in support of a model that predicts how biological and environmental factors interact to influence spatial skills. *Dev Psychol, 35*, 1237-1247.

[12] Cohen, M.S., Kosslyn, S. M., Breiter, H. C., DiGirolamo, G. J., Thompson, W. L., Anderson, A., K.Brookheimer, S. Y., Rosen, B. R., and Belliveau, J. W. (1996). Changes in cortical activity during mental rotation. A mapping study using functional MRI. *Brain, 119 (Pt 1)*, 89-100.

[13] Cooper, L., and Shepard ,R. (1973). The time required to prepare for a rotated stimulus. *Mem Cognit, 1*, 246-250.

[14] Corballis, M.C. (1997). Mental rotation and the right hemisphere. *Brain Lang, 57*, 100-121.

[15] de Lange, F.P., Hagoort, P., and Toni, I. (2005). Neural topography and content of movement representations, *J Cogn Neurosci, 17*, 97-112.

[16] de Lange, F.P., Helmich, R.C., and Toni, I. (2006). Posture influences motor imagery: an fMRI study. *Neuroimage, 33*, 609-61.

[17] Ditunno, P.L., and Mann, V.A., (1990). Right hemisphere specialization for mental rotation in normals and brain damaged subjects. *Cortex, 26*, 177-188.

[18] Eley, M.G. (1982). Identifying rotated letter-like symbols. *Mem Cognit, 10*, 25-32.

[19] Feredoes, E. A., and Sachdev, P. S. (2006). Differential effects of transcranial magnetic stimulation of left and right posterior parietal cortex on mental rotation tasks. *Cortex, 42*, 750-754.

[20] Funk, M., and Brugger, P. (2008). Mental rotation of congenitally absent hands. *J Int Neuropsychol Soc, 14*, 81-89.

[21] Ganis, G., Keenan, J. P., Kosslyn, S. M., and Pascual-Leone, A. (2000). Transcranial magnetic stimulation of primary motor cortex affects mental rotation. *Cereb Cortex, 10*, 175-180.

[22] Gentilucci, M., Daprati, E., and Gangitano, M. (1998). Right-handers and left-handers have different representations of their own hand. *Brain Res Cogn Brain Res, 6*, 185-192.

[23] Geschwind, N., and Galaburda, A.M. (1985). Cerebral lateralization. Biological mechanisms, associations, and pathology: I. A hypothesis and a program for research. *Arch Neurol, 42*, 428-459.

[24] Gonzalez, C.L., Whitwell, R. L., Morrissey, B., Ganel, T., and Goodale, M. A. (2007). Left handedness does not extend to visually guided precision grasping. *Exp Brain Res, 182*, 275-279.

[25] Gur, R.C., Ragland, J. D., Resnick, S. M., Skolnick, B. E., Jaggi, J., Muenz, L., and Gur, R. E. (1994). Lateralized increases in cerebral blood flow during performance of verbal and spatial tasks: relationship with performance level. *Brain Cogn, 24*, 244-258.

[26] Harris, I.M., Egan, G. F., Sonkkila, C., Tochon-Danguy, H. J., Paxinos, G., and Watson, J. D. (2000). Selective right parietal lobe activation during mental rotation: a parametric PET study. *Brain, 123 (Pt 1)*, 65-73.

[27] Hecaen, H., De Agostini, M., and Monzon-Montes, A. (1981). Cerebral organization in left-handers. *Brain Lang, 12*, 261-284.

[28] Helmich, R.C., de Lange, F. P., Bloem, B. R., and Toni, I. (2007). Cerebral compensation during motor imagery in Parkinson's disease. *Neuro-psychologia, 45*, 2201-2215.

[29] Herrmann, D.J., and van Dyke, K.A. (1978). Handedness and the mental rotation of perceived patterns. *Cortex, 14,* 521-529.

[30] Ionta, S., Fourkas, A. D., Fiorio, M., and Aglioti, S. M. (2007). The influence of hands posture on mental rotation of hands and feet. Exp *Brain Res, 183*, 1-7.

[31] Ionta, S., and Blanke O. (2009). Differential influence of hands posture on mental rotation of hands and feet in left and right handers. *Exp Brain Res, 195*, 207-217.

[32] Jäncke, L., and Jordan, K. (2007). Functional neuroanatomy of mental rotation performance. In Mast F. W. Editor, and Jäncke L. Editor, Spatial Processing in Navigation, Imagery and Perception. (pp.183-207). New York, Springer.

[33] Jeannerod, M., and Decety, J. (1995). Mental motor imagery: a window into the representational stages of action. *Curr Opin Neurobiol, 5*, 727-732.

[34] Johnson, B.W., McKenzie, K.J., and Hamm, J.P. (2002). Cerebral asymmetry for mental rotation: effects of response hand, handedness and gender. *Neuroreport, 13*, 1929-1932.

[35] Jones, B., and Anuza T. (1982). Effects of sex, handedness, stimulus and visual field on "mental rotation". *Cortex, 18*, 501-514.

[36] Jordan, K., Wustenberg, T., Heinze, H. J., Peters, M., and Jancke, L. (2002). Women and men exhibit different cortical activation patterns during mental rotation tasks. *Neuropsychologia, 40*, 2397-2408.

[37] Kawamichi, H., Kikuchi, Y., Endo, H., Takeda, T., and Yoshizawa, S. (1998). Temporal structure of implicit motor imagery in visual hand-shape discrimination as revealed by MEG. *Neuroreport, 9*, 1127-1132.

[38] Kilshaw, D., and Annett, M. (1983). Right- and left-hand skill I: Effects of age, sex and hand preference showing superior skill in left-handers. *Br J Psychol, 74 (Pt 2)*.253-268.

[39] Kimberley, T. J., Khandekar, G., Skraba, L. L., Spencer, J. A., Van Gorp, E. A., and Walker, S. R. (2006). Neural substrates for motor imagery in severe hemiparesis. *Neurorehabil Neural Repair, 20*, 268-277.

[40] Kosslyn, S.M., DiGirolamo, G. J., Thompson, W. L., and Alpert, N. M. (1998). Mental rotation of objects versus hands: neural mechanisms revealed by positron emission tomography. *Psychophysiology, 35*, 151-161.

[41] Lewis, R.S., and Harris, L.J. (1990). Handedness, Sex, and Spatial Ability. In Coren S.Editor, Left-Handedness: Behavioral Implication and Anomalies. (pp.319-341). New York, North-Holland.

[42] Li, C., Zhu, W., and Nuttall, R.L. (2003). Familial handedness and spatial ability: a study with Chinese students aged 14-24. *Brain Cogn, 51*, 375-384.

[43] Maki, A., Yamashita, Y., Ito, Y., Watanabe, E., Mayanagi, Y. and Koizumi, H. (1995). Spatial and temporal analysis of human motor activity using noninvasive NIR topography. *Med Phys, 22*, 1997-2005.

[44] Maruff, P., Wilson, P. H., De Fazio, J., Cerritelli, B., Hedt, A., and Currie, J. (1999). Asymmetries between dominant and non-dominant hands in real and imagined motor task performance. *Neuropsychologia, 37*, 379-384.

[45] McGee, M.G. (1978). Handedness and mental rotation. *Percept Mot Skills, 47*, 641-642.

[46] Moseley, G.L. (2004). Graded motor imagery is effective for long-standing complex regional pain syndrome: a randomised controlled trial. *Pain, 108*, 192-198.

[47] Mutsaarts, M., Steenbergen, B., and Bekkering, H. (2007). Impaired motor imagery in right hemiparetic cerebral palsy. *Neuropsychologia, 45*, 853-859.

[48] Nico, D., Daprati, E., Rigal, F., Parsons, L., and Sirigu, A. (2004). Left and right hand recognition in upper limb amputees. *Brain, 127*, 120-132.

[49] Oldfield, R. C. (1971). The assessment and analysis of handedness: the Edinburgh inventory. *Neuropsychologia, 9*, 97-113.

[50] Page, S. J., Levine, P., Sisto, S., and Johnston, M. V. (2001). A randomized efficacy and feasibility study of imagery in acute stroke. *Clin Rehabil, 15*, 233-240.

[51] Parsons, L.M. (1987). Imagined spatial transformations of one's hands and feet. *Cognit Psychol, 19*, 178-241.

[52] Parsons, L. M. (1994). Temporal and kinematic properties of motor behavior reflected in mentally simulated action. *J Exp Psychol Hum Percept Perform, 20*, 709-730.

[53] Parsons, L.M., Fox, P. T., Downs, J. H., Glass, T., Hirsch, T. B., Martin, C. C., Jerabek, P. A., and Lancaster, J. L. (1995). Use of implicit motor imagery for visual shape discrimination as revealed by PET. *Nature, 375*, 54-58.

[54] Peters, M., Laeng, B., Latham, K., Jackson, M., Zaiyouna, R., and Richardson, C. (1995). A redrawn Vandenberg and Kuse mental rotations test: different versions and factors that affect performance. *Brain Cogn, 28*, 39-58.

[55] Pezaris, E., and Casey, M.B. (1991). Girls who use "masculine" problem-solving strategies on a spatial task: proposed genetic and environmental factors. *Brain Cogn, 17*, 1-22.

[56] Rumiati, R.I., Tomasino, B., Vorano, L., Umilta, C., and De Luca, G. (2001). Selective deficit of imagining finger configurations. *Cortex, 37*, 730-733.

[57] Sanders, B., Wilson, J.R., and Vandenberg, S.G. (1982). Handedness and spatial ability. *Cortex, 18*, 79-89.

[58] Sauner, D., Bestmann, S., Siebner, H. R. and Rothwell, J. C. (2006) No evidence for a substantial involvement of primary motor hand area in handedness judgements: a transcranial magnetic stimulation study. *Eur J Neurosci, 23*, 2215-2224.

[59] Sekiyama, K. (1982). Kinesthetic aspects of mental representations in the identification of left and right hands. *Percept Psychophys, 32*, 89-95.

[60] Seurinck, R., Vingerhoets, G.,Vandemaele, P., Deblaere, K., and Achten, E. (2005). Trial pacing in mental rotation tasks. *Neuroimage, 25*, 1187-1196.

[61] Sherman, J. (1978). Sex-related cognitive difference. Springfield, IL: Charles C. Thomas.

[62] Sheehan, E.P., and Smith, H.V. (1986). Cerebral lateralization and handedness and their effects on verbal and spatial reasoning. *Neuropsychologia, 24*, 531-540.

[63] Shepard, R.N., and Metzler, J. (1971). Mental rotation of three-dimensional objects. *Science, 171*, 701-703.

[64] Shimoda, N., Takeda, K., Imai, I., Kaneko, J., and Kato, H. (2008). Cerebral laterality differences in handedness: a mental rotation study with NIRS. *Neurosci Lett, 430*, 43-47.

[65] Snyder, P.J., and Harris, L.J. (1993). Handedness, sex, and familial sinistrality effects on spatial tasks. *Cortex, 29*, 115-134.

[66] Steenbergen, B., van Nimwegen, M., and Craje, C. (2007). Solving a mental rotation task in congenital hemiparesis: motor imagery versus visual imagery. *Neuropsychologia, 45*, 3324-3328.

[67] Szaflarski, J.P., Binder, J. R., Possing, E. T., McKiernan, K. A., Ward, B. D., and Hammeke, T. A. (2002). Language lateralization in left-handed and ambidextrous people: fMRI data. *Neurology, 59*, 238-244.

[68] Takeda, K., Gomi, Y., Imai, I., Shimoda, N., Hiwatari, M., and Kato, H.(2007). Shift of motor activation areas during recovery from hemiparesis after cerebral infarction: A longitudinal study with near-infrared spectroscopy. *Neurosci Res, 59*, 136-144.

[69] Takeda, K., Shimoda, N., Sato, Y., Ogano, M., and Kato, H. (2009). Reaction time differences between left- and right-handers during mental rotation of hand pictures. *Laterality 14*, 415-425.

[70] Thayer, Z.C., and Johnson, B.W., (2006). Cerebral processes during visuo-motor imagery of hands. *Psychophysiology, 43*, 401-412.

[71] Thomsen, T., Hugdahl, K., Ersland, L., Barndon, R., Lundervold, A., Smievoll, A. I., Roscher, B. E., and Sundberg, H. (2000). Functional magnetic resonance imaging (fMRI) study of sex differences in a mental rotation task. *Med Sci Monit, 6*, 1186-1196.

[72] Tomasino, B., Toraldo, A., and Rumiati, R.I., (2003). Dissociation between the mental rotation of visual images and motor images in unilateral brain-damaged patients. *Brain Cogn, 51*, 368-371.

[73] Tomasino, B., Borroni, P., Isaja, A., and Rumiati, R. I. (2005). The role of the primary motor cortex in mental rotation: a TMS study. *Cogn Neuropsychol, 22*, 348-363.

[74] Vandenberg, S. G., and Kuse, A. R. (1978). Mental rotations, a group test of three-dimensional spatial visualization. *Percept Mot Skills, 47*, 599-604.

[75] Van Strien, J.W., Licht, R., Bouma, A., and Bakker, D. J. (1989). Event-related potentials during word-reading and figure-matching in left-handed and right-handed males and females. *Brain Lang, 37*, 525-547.

[76] Voyer, D., and Bryden, M.P., (1990). Gender, level of spatial ability, and lateralization of mental rotation. *Brain Cogn, 13*, 18-29.

[77] Voyer, D., Voyer, S., and Bryden, M.P., (1995). Magnitude of sex differences in spatial abilities: a meta-analysis and consideration of critical variables. *Psychol Bull, 117*, 250-270.

[78] Weiss, E., Siedentopf, C. M., Hofer, A., Deisenhammer, E. A., Hoptman, M. J., Kremser, C., Golaszewski, S., Felber, S., Fleischhacker, W. W., and Delazer, M. (2003). Sex differences in brain activation pattern during a visuospatial cognitive task: a functional magnetic resonance imaging study in healthy volunteers. *Neurosci Lett, 344*, 169-172.

[79] Wisniewski, A.B., Prendeville, M.T., and Dobs, A.S. (2005). Handedness, functional cerebral hemispheric lateralization, and cognition in male-to-female transsexuals receiving cross-sex hormone treatment. *Arch Sex Behav, 34*, 167-172.

[80] Zacks, J.M. (2008). Neuroimaging studies of mental rotation: a meta-analysis and review. *J Cogn Neurosci, 20*, 1-19.

[81] A part of this article was supported by SRBPS, MEXT, and CREST, JST.

In: Handedness: Theories, Genetics and Psychology ISBN: 978-1-61470-502-4
Editors: J. Dunham and T. Davenport

Chapter V

Left, Right, Hand `n Space

Michael J. Banissy[1], Lucy E. Annett[2], Patience Asiedu-Offei[2], Richard Rosch[3] and Jennifer M. Gurd[4,*]

[1]Institute of Cognitive Neuroscience, University College London, UK
[2]School of Psychology, University of Hertfordshire, Hatfield, UK
[3]Magdalen College Oxford, UK
[4]Nuffield Department of Clinical Neurosciences (Clinical Neurology), University of Oxford, UK

Abstract

A finger tapping task was employed to investigate fine motor performance rate by healthy adult right (RH) and left (LH) handers in right versus left hemispace. Eighty healthy adults tapped rapidly with the right or left hand index finger during uncued, unpaced, uni- and bimanual conditions. Two strikingly significant results emerged: (1.) The right hand showed a significant effect of space, but the left hand did not; this irrespective of handedness or number of hands employed. (2.) This effect of space favoured the right side. Overall, these findings support fMRI and lesion evidence

* Corresponding author. University Nuffield Department of Clinical Neurosciences (Clinical Neurology) , The John Radcliffe Hospital West Wing, Oxford, OX3 9DU, UK. Email address: jennifer.gurd@clneuro.ox.ac.uk.

indicating that side of space influences the extent of motor asymmetry. The result is novel and shows an effect which is independent of hand preference; that is, right versus left handedness.

Keywords: Attention, Cerebral laterality, Finger tapping, Handedness, Motor control, Motor performance, Tapping space

1. Introduction

A notable characteristic of the brain is the functional asymmetry between left and right cerebral hemispheres (Marshall and Fink, 2003; Stephan et al., 2007). To some degree, cerebral asymmetries are found to be reflected by behavioural measures - an everyday example of which is *handedness* (Lutz et al., 2005). The term *handedness* can refer to two phenomena. One is the seemingly inherent preference of individuals for using a particular hand to perform certain tasks. The hand *preference* component of handedness is frequently represented as a continuously distributed (versus discrete) variable (cf. Gurd et al., 2006), which can be assessed through questionnaires such as the Handedness Preference Inventory (HPI) (Gurd et al., 2006; Oldfield, 1971) and which taps a range of everyday tasks (Annett, 1967; Corey et al., 2001). Additionally, *handedness* encompasses some degree of performance difference between the hands. Tasks used to assess hand *performance* (e.g. dot filling, finger tapping, peg moving) quantify relative manual rate and accuracy with each hand (Annett, 1972; Gurd et al., 2006; Tapley and Bryden, 1985; Nalçaci et al., 2001). Performance tasks also vary in terms of degree of skill and practice involved (Hausmann et al., 2004). Thus, differences in the performance of left and right hands tend to be discussed in the context of underlying motor asymmetries (e.g. Annett, 2002). (Annett and colleagues (Annett, 1985) have claimed that there is a factor which yields hand performance result distributions displaced to the right, in association with cerebral asymmetry favouring left hemisphere dominance, but this view is not without controversy (cf. Keane,1999).)

One overlooked factor is that laterality of hand performance effects may be confounded by hemispace, since each hand is more likely to be used in its ipsilateral hemispace. Furthermore, cerebral visuospatial attentional circuits are asymmetrically organised, such that left and right hemispace are represented differently (Bottini et al., 2010). In principle, it has been unclear whether motor laterality factors predominate over visuo-spatial ones (cf. Aramaki et al., 2006; Graziano and Taylor, 2002; Gut et al., 2007; Verstynen et al., 2005; Yamamoto and Kitazawa, 2001), and if so, under what conditions. And yet, the influence of hemispace on overall hand preference and performance differences (and thus *handedness*), has not yet been investigated experimentally. The study reported here includes hemispace as an experimental variable by measuring tapping rate of each hand in its respective ipsilateral or contralateral side of body-centred space. Comparing right (RH) and left handers (LH), the study is designed to identify the effects of hemispace, independent of hand preference. If hemispace is an independent factor, then its effects on right or left hand performance, in right versus left space would be similar in RH and LH individuals (cf. Witt et al., 2008).

2. Method

2.1. Participants

Eighty adults (RH: N=40; LH: N=40) participated in the study. One male subject who wrote with his left hand but scored as a right hander (HPI: +61.9), was removed from the analysis. Likewise, one left handed female, and two right handed males with excessively high or low outlying tapping scores (+/- 2 SD), were also removed from the analysis. Data from 19 female LH and 19 male LH (mean age = 23.2 years, SEM ± 1.1), and 20 female RH and 18 male RH (mean age = 24.1, SEM ± 1.2) participants were retained. (Ethics approval was granted by the University of Hertfordshire Psychology Department Ethics panel.)

2.2. Materials and Procedures

The modified Hand Preference Inventory (HPI) (Gurd et al., 2006), composed of 16 items from the Briggs and Nebes (1975) and Edinburgh Handedness Inventories (Oldfield, 1971) was completed as a pencil and paper task prior to experimental testing. For each item subjects responded either: *always right* (+2), *usually right* (+1), *no preference* (0), *usually left (-1)*, or *always left* (-2). The total HPI scores were calculated by dividing the sum of the scores by the maximum (i.e. 32), and multiplying by 100, providing scores ranging from -100 (strongly left handed) to +100 (strongly right handed). Based on the HPI scores, participants were grouped as either LH (≤ 0) or RH (≥ 0) (Corey et al., 2001; Gurd et al., 2006).

The experimental finger tapping task employed a custom designed tapping board, 43 cm (w) by 26.5 cm (d) containing two buttons; one was 8.5 cm in from the edge of the board on the left side, and the other 8.5 cm in from the edge on the right side. The board was attached to a computer which recorded the number of taps (per ten second interval). Participants were seated at a table on which the button board was located in front of them and at their midline. They were instructed to tap on the button as quickly as possible using the index finger (with eyes open). It was explained that the computer would begin to measure tap frequency following the first button press. Tapping was self-paced and un-cued, with no feedback provided. Participants commenced the task with either the preferred or non-preferred hand, in either ipsilateral (i.e. arms uncrossed), or contralateral (i.e. arms crossed) space. This order was counter-balanced across all subjects. Following the first trial, participants switched to using the other hand, in the other side of space. This alternation was repeated until each hand had been tested 5 times per condition. Participants performed 5 alternating trials with each hand, in each condition (i.e. if the hands had been uncrossed previously, they were then crossed, or *vice versa*). In addition to unimanual (i.e. one hand tapping), participants were also tested bimanually, using both hands simultaneously. Thus, preferred and non-preferred hands were employed both in ipsilateral and contralateral space (i.e. either the right hand pressed the button which was in right hemispace while the left hand pressed the button in left hemispace, or the right hand pressed the button which was in left hemispace while the left hand pressed the button in right hemispace). Again, five trials per condition alternated between the two conditions with the start condition counter-balanced across subjects.

3. Results

3.1. Hand Preference

The HPI scores were LH: (N=38) mean = -69.1 (SEM ± 3.2; range -100 to -3.2), and RH: (N=38) mean = +86.0 (SEM ± 2.3; range +34.4 to +100.0).

3.2. Finger Tapping

Finger tapping rate (number of taps per 10 seconds) was analysed using a 2 *(handedness: RH, LH)* x 2 *(hand used: right hand, left hand)* x 2 *(hemispace:*

right hemispace, left hemispace) analysis of variance (ANOVA). Unimanual condition results are presented first (Figure 1a, 1b), followed by bimanual ones (Figure 1c, 1d). The dependent variable was number of taps in 10 seconds.

3.2.1. Uni-manual Performance

There were no overall significant main effects of *hand used,* or of *handedness* group on the unimanual conditions. However, there was a significant interaction between *hand used* and *handedness* group ($F(1,74) = 90.46$, $p < .001$), due to the greater number of taps produced by the preferred hand for both groups (RH: *hand used*, $F(1,37) = 47.95$, $p < .001$; LH: *hand used,* $F(1,37) = 42.59$, $p < .001$). Of particular note is the finding that overall performance in right hemispace was significantly greater than in left hemispace ($F(1,74) = 18.97$, $p < .001$; right hemispace mean = 57.92, SEM ± 1.00; left hemispace mean = 55.97, SEM ± 1.11). The interaction between *hand used* and *hemispace* was also significant ($F(1,74) = 18.83$, $p < .001$), due to the increased right hand performance rate when in right (versus left) (mean = 55.03, SEM ± 1.19), hemispace (mean = 59.29, SEM ± 1.03). However, the left hand performance was equally good in right (versus left) (mean = 56.56, SEM ± 1.08), hemispace (mean = 56.92, SEM ± 1.16). The right versus left hand difference in right versus left hemispace was evident for both the RH and LH groups. Thus, the interaction of *handedness* x *hand used* x *hemispace* was *not* significant ($F(1,74) = .34$, ns). Within group comparisons for each hand revealed that the RH group showed a significant increase when performing with the right hand in right, versus left hemispace ($F(1,37) = 13.19$, $p < .01$). The LH group also showed a significant right hand decrease in left versus right hemispace ($F(1,37) = 16.92$, $p < .001$). In contrast, no significant differences were found for either handedness group when tapping with the left hand in right versus left hemispace (RH: *hemispace*, $F(1,37) = .35$, ns; LH: *hemispace*, $F(1,37) = .09$, ns) (Figure 1a, 1b).

The RH group showed greater uncrossed asymmetry than did the LH group (i.e. right hand in right hemispace and left hand in left hemispace). By contrast, this asymmetry was reversed when the hands were crossed (i.e. right hand in left hemispace and left hand in right hemispace), such that between-hand differences were greater for the LH versus RH. The differences were confirmed by further ANOVAs; performance with the preferred versus non-preferred hands was compared in uncrossed and crossed conditions (i.e. 3 factor ANOVA, 2 *(handedness: RH, LH)* x 2 *(hand used: preferred, non-preferred)* x 2 *(condition: uncrossed, crossed)*). The interaction *handedness* x *preferred/non-preferred hand* x *uncrossed/crossed* was significant ($F(1,74) = 18.97$, $p < .001$). With respect to uncrossed performance only, the interaction *handedness* x *preferred/non-*

preferred hand was significant (F (1,74) = 13.90, $p < .001$); this was due to the greater asymmetry shown by the RH (right hand mean = 61.04, SEM ± 1.45; left hand mean = 53.87, SEM ± 1.61; t = 8.92, df 37, $p < .001$), versus the LH (right hand mean = 57.54, SEM ± 1.45; left hand mean = 59.97, SEM ± 1.68; t = 2.47, df 37, $p = .018$) groups. For crossed performance, the interaction *handedness* x *preferred/non-preferred hand* was also significant (F (1,74) = 5.02, $p < .05$), but this was due to the greater asymmetry for the LH (right hand mean = 53.77, SEM ± 1.60; left hand mean = 59.73, SEM ± 1.60; t = 7.65, df 37, $p < .001$) versus the RH (right hand mean = 56.28, SEM ± 1.77; left hand mean = 53.39, SEM ± 1.45; t = 2.57, df 37, $p = .014$) group.

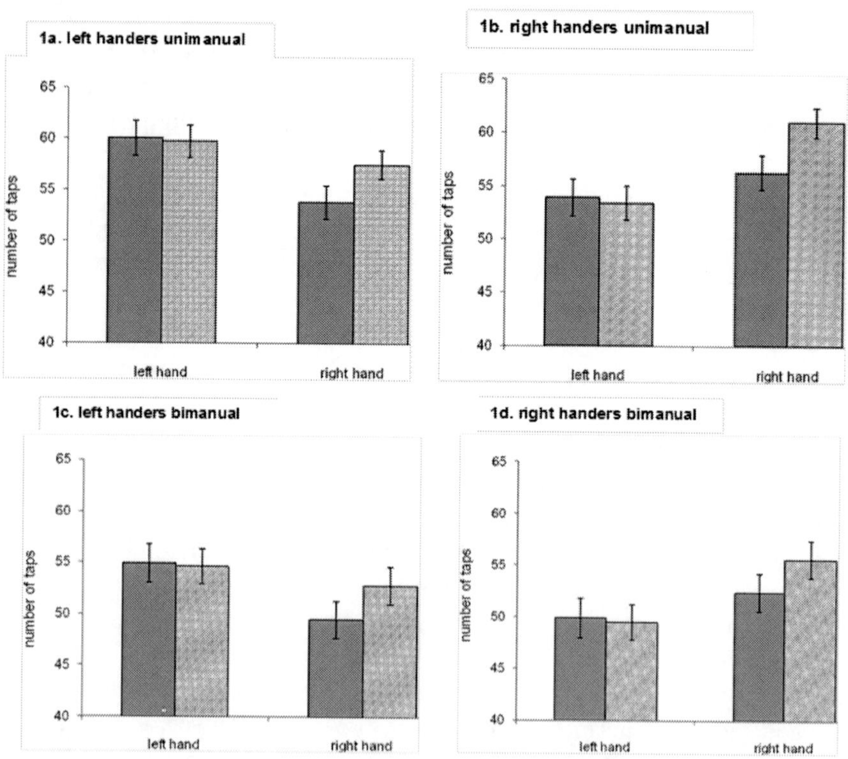

Figure 1. Mean number of taps/ 10 sec trial for LH (1a, 1c), and RH (1b, 1d), using the index finger of the *right* or *left* hand, in *right* or *left* hemispace; unimanual (1a, 1b), bimanual (1c, 1d), (error bars represent +/- SEM).

3.2.2. Bimanual Performance

When the finger tapping task was performed bi-manually, the pattern of results resembled the unimanual ones, although fewer taps were made overall (F (1,74) = 83.54, $p < .001$). There were no significant main effects of *hand used,* or of *handedness*. The interaction between *hand used* and *handedness* was significant (F (1,74) = 43.09, $p < .001$), indicating that in both handedness groups, more taps were produced with the preferred (versus non-preferred) hand (RH: *hand used*, F (1,37) = 26.71, $p < .001$; LH: *hand used,* F(1,37) = 17.11, $p < .001$).

A significant main effect of *hemispace* was again found (F (1,74) = 8.30, $p < .01$), with participants producing more taps in right (mean = 53.13, SEM ± 1.13), versus left hemispace (mean = 51.67, SEM ± 1.17). There was also a significant interaction between *hand used* and *hemispace* (F (1,74) = 9.07, $p < .01$). This was due to the difference in right hand performance in left (mean = 50.93, SEM ± 1.24), versus right hemispace (mean = 54.23, SEM ± 1.24); although left hand performance was equally good in left (mean = 52.40, SEM ± 1.30), versus right hemispace (mean = 52.04, SEM ± 1.24).

The interaction *handedness x hand used x hemispace* was not significant for bimanual taps (F (1,74) = .004, ns). Within-group comparisons for each hand showed a significant difference for RH performance with the right hand tapping in left, versus right hemispace (F (1,37) = 6.42, $p < .05$); and for LH performance with the right hand in left versus right hemispace (F (1,37) = 7.77, $p < .01$). Again, no significant differences were found for either group using the left hand in right, or in left hemispace (RH: *hemispace*, F (1,37) = .145, ns; LH: *hemispace,* F (1,37) = .128, ns). Therefore, as was the case for the unimanual conditions, both RH and LH showed a difference in right hand performance when tapping in right (faster) versus left (slower) hemispace (Figure 1c, 1d).

Thus, the greater asymmetry in the RH group when tapping with hands uncrossed was as evident bimanually as it was unimanually. When the hands were crossed bimanually, the LH group showed greater asymmetry (*handedness* x *preferred/non-preferred hand* x *uncrossed/crossed,* F (1,74) = 8.30, $p <.01$). With respect to bimanual performance with hands uncrossed (only), the interaction *handedness* x *preferred/non-preferred hand* was significant (F (1,74) = 5.94, $p < .05$); this is due to the greater asymmetry of the RH (RH: mean = 55.62, SEM ± 1.82; LH: mean = 49.86, SEM ± 1.77; t = 5.11, df 37, $p < .001$), versus the LH (right hand mean = 52.84, SEM ± 1.77; left hand mean = 54.94, SEM ± 1.82; t = 2.12, df 37, $p = .04$). With the hands crossed bimanually, the asymmetry shown by the RH group decreased (right hand mean = 52.37, SEM = 1.69; left hand mean = 49.53, SEM ± 1.82; t = 2.36, df 37, $p = .024$), whereas that shown by the LH group increased (right hand mean = 49.50, SEM ± 1.82; left hand mean =

54.55, SEM = 1.69; t = 4.52, df 37, $p < .001$), although the interaction *handedness* x *preferred/non-preferred hand* with the hands crossed (only) bimanually, did not reach statistical significance (F (1,74) = 1.81, $p = .18$).

Discussion

The results presented here bear testimony to the view that: "Handedness (...) is an asymmetry that depends not on structural asymmetry of the hands themselves, but rather on cerebral asymmetry" (Corballis, 2008, p. 4). The most striking effect we demonstrate is the advantage of right space. Hence, the side of space in which actions are performed *does* influence the extent of the motor asymmetry. Witt et al. (2008) conducted a meta-analysis of the neural systems involved in a variety of finger tapping tasks. The cortical networks included: primary sensorimotor cortices, supplementary motor area, premoter, inferior parietal, basal ganglia, and anterior cerebellum. It is likely that the attentional role of the inferior parietal cortical regions and their connections via the ventral stream systems involved in the generation and recognition of sets of actions (Arbib, 2006), are particularly salient to the right hand performing in right space. That is, because the right hand is controlled by the left hemisphere, and the left hemisphere attends preferentially to right space, the right hand is advantaged when tapping in right space (cf. Serrien et al., 2003; 2008)). It follows that since the left hand is controlled by the right hemisphere, and the right hemisphere attends to both sides of space, the left hand is *not* advantaged in right space. Thus, over and above any left hemisphere dominance for finger tapping (Pollock et al., 2006; 2008; Rogalsky et al., 2008), the additive effects of tapping space are also demonstrably significant.

To elaborate, it is the added right space attentional component which confers the cumulative effect, because if only balanced contralateral effects were salient, then the two sides of space would receive equal attentional balance. That *added* right sided component is conferred by the right hemisphere contribution to parietal lobe circuits (cf. Chokron, 2003; Marshall and Fink, 2003; Passingham and Toni, 2001; Rushworth et al., 2003). Evidence converges on inferior parietal components of neural activity associated with finger tapping performance (Witt et al., 2008). Corbetta's group (Shulman et al., 2010) have shown this to be attributed to detection of relevant stimuli which is by their account, a right hemisphere component (Arbib, 2006; Bottini et al., 2010). This effect is independent of handedness preference as shown here.

Several qualifications are apposite. (a.) It is important to emphasize that our finger tapping results are limited to simple unskilled actions, and that skilled actions might produce different patterns of results (Haaland et al., 2004; Hausmann et al., 2004). (b.) With respect to practice effects, we make no specific empirically based claims (cf. Koeneke et al., 2006). Although we assume that (from an ecological point of view) finger tapping is a practiced task in our population (cf. Gurd et al., 2006), practice effects *per se* were not subjected to experimental manipulation (cf. Gerloff and Andres, 2002). Delineating implications for functional cerebral laterality via deficit analysis studies of brain damage have tended to focus on more complex tasks (Calautti and Baron, 2003; Cramer et al., 2001; Haaland et al., 2004; Verstynen et al., 2005; Witt et al., 2008)), for which the mechanisms and neural circuitry no doubt differ from tapping. (c.) It is notable that as a group, the left handers differed from the right handers with respect to heterogeneity (larger ranges and variances than the RH), and therefore the LH could also be named `mixed', or `non-right' handed.

In future research the functional and structural connections between attention, perception, and executive processes salient to simple finger tapping warrant further investigation. In principle, we are able to show the significance of asymmetric visuospatial attention implicit in this motor task, but there are several possibilities as to how this could arise (e.g. via parietal networks involved in motor execution (Pisella, 2000), and cerebellar loops involved in visuospatial attention and motor tasks (Ramnani, 2006)). (Although it would have been ideal, eye movements were not measured here, due to technical constraints.) Characterising how different motor tasks are differentially influenced by the hemispace in which they are performed, could aid in detailing the full extent of the underlying neural networks involved and their respective mechanisms (cf. Bundesen and Habekost, 2008; Karnath et al., 2002).

There is a broader significance to these findings, pertaining to theories of brain development, since one fundamental question about laterality focuses on cause and effect. In this case, the effect of practice is independent from whatever has caused hand preference. That is, assuming that finger tapping is a fundamentally practiced, as opposed to novel task, then this long term practiced relationship to attentional hemispace laterality differences is unlikely to be a causal one. Put differently, space-motor laterality effects appear to be independent of handedness preference laterality, precluding strong causal effects of task-specific experience on visuospatial attention. This is not to imply that environmental effects of living in a right-handers' world play no significant effect, merely that the factors are separable. It would be a separate question to ask what the impact of interaction with objects on the right side of space would be on the development of cortical circuits for hemi-spatial attention. It is pertinent to unpack our *lack* of significant added bimanual effects, since these would be more likely to reflect a potential callosal component indicative of practice effects, given that increased thickening of the corpus callosum (Yoon et al., 2010), has been associated with increased practice effects at different ages during development (cf. Haberling et al., 2011). The lack of evidence pointing to such effects in our results may weigh the balance of interpretation in favour of laterality effects originating in visuospatial attentional differences, rather than vice-versa (if there *is* a causal effect to be postulated). This line of argument is congruent with current results from functional imaging and lesion studies which broadly show that the left hemisphere controls the right hand and also confers *added* attentional bias to the right side of body-centred visual space (Arbib, 2006; Bottini et al., 2010; Fink et al., 2001). Our group (Rosch et al., 2010a, 2010b; Lux et al., 2008) has also shown that in the lack of a strongly lateralised right hemisphere parietal contribution to visuospatial attention, such effects can be comparatively skewed even further into right space overall (particularly when performing with the right hand), and this even in a strongly left-handed person. In evolutionary terms therefore, it seems unlikely that handedness preference came first.

Conclusion

The way in which the right and left hands reference (and are referenced by) space, is different. It impacts on performance such that greater attention to right space confers an advantage (or conversely, lesser attending to left space confers a comparative disadvantage). This pertains to visuospatial contributions to simple finger tapping tasks; fine motor manual unskilled, uncued, speeded, continuous, unpaced performance in body-centred space.

Acknowledgment

We are grateful to: M. and J. Annett for comments on the manuscript, M. Rawlings for the apparatus, J. Schulz for statistics, J. Critchley, The British Academy, and the Medical Research Council (UK) for financial support, and to G. Ebers, G.R. Fink, and J.C. Marshall (deceased) for contributions to the research. We are grateful to Dr P Cowell for referees' comments on the manuscript.

References

Annett M. (1967). The binomial distribution of right, mixed and left handedness. *Quarterly Journal of Experimental Psychology, 19*, 327-333.

Annett M. (1972). The distribution of manual asymmetry. *British Journal of Psychology, 63,* 343-358.

Annett M. (1985). *Left, right, hand, brain: The right shift theory.* Hove, UK: Lawrence Erlbaum Associates.

Annett M. (2002). *Handedness and brain asymmetry: The right shift theory.* Hove, East Sussex: Psychology Press.

Aramiki, Y., Honda, M., and Sadato, N. (2006). Suppression of the non-dominant motor cortex during bimanual symmetric finger movement: A functional magnetic resonance imaging study. *Neuroscience, 141*, 2147-2153.

Arbib, M. (2006). Broca's area in system perspective: Language in the context of action-oriented perception. In: Y. Grozinsky and K. Amunts (Eds.) *Broca's Region*. Oxford, UK: Oxford University Press, pp. 153-168.

Bottini, G., Paulesu, P., Gandola, M. and Invernizzi, P. (2010). Functional neuroanatomy of spatial perception, spatial processes and attention. In: J.M.Gurd, U. Kischka and J.C. Marshall (Eds.) *Handbook of Clinical Neuropsychology*, 2nd Edition. Oxford, UK: Oxford University Press, pp. 765-792.

Briggs, G.G., and Nebes, R.D. (1975). Patterns of hand preference in a student population. *Cortex, 11,* 230-238.

Bundesen, C., and Habekost, T. (2008). *Principles of Visual Attention: Linking Mind And Brain*. Oxford, UK: Oxford University Press.

Calautti, C., and Baron, J-C. (2003). Functional neuroimaging studies of motor recovery after stroke in adults: a review. *Stroke*, *34,* 1553-1566.

Chokron, S. (2003). Right parietal lesions, unilateral spatial neglect, and the egocentric frame of reference. *NeuroImage, 20*, S75-S81.

Cramer, S.C., Nelles, G., Schaechter, J.D., Kaplan, J.D., Finklestein, S.P., and Rosen, B.R. (2001). A functional MRI study of three motor tasks in the evaluation of stroke recovery. *Neurorehabilitation Neural Repair*, *15*, 1-8.

Corballis, M. (2008). Of mice and men – and lopsided birds. *Cortex, 44*, 3-7.

Corey, D.M., Hurley, M., and Foundas, A. (2001). Right and left handedness defined. *Neuropsychiatry, Neuropsychology and Behavioural Neurology*, *14*, 144-152.

Fink, G.R., Marshall, J.C., Weiss, P.H. and Zilles, K. (2001). The neural basis of vertical and horizontal line bisection judgments: An fMRI Study of normal volunteers. *NeuroImage, 14*, S59-S67.

Gerloff, C., and Andres, F.G. (2002). Bimanual coordination and interhemispheric interaction. *Acta Psychologica*, *110,* 161-186.

Graziano, M.S.A., and Taylor, C.S.R. (2002). The cortical control of movement revisited. *Neuron, 36,* 349-362.

Gurd, J.M., Schulz, J., Cherkas, L., and Ebers, G.C. (2006). Hand preference and performance in 20 pairs of monozygotic twins with discordant handedness. *Cortex*, *42*, 934-945.

Gut, M., Urbanik, A., Forsberg, L., Binder, M., Rymarczyk, K., Sobiecka, B., Kozub, J., and Grabowska, A. (2007). Brain correlates of right-handedness. *Acta Neurobiologiae Experimentalis, 67,* 43-51.

Haaland, K.Y., Elsinger, C.L., Mayer, A.R., Durgerian, S., and Rao, S.M. (2004). Motor sequence complexity and performing hand produce differential patterns of hemispheric lateralization. *Journal of Cognitive Neuroscience, 16,* 621-636.

Haberling, I.S., Badzakova-Trajkov, G., and Corballis, M.C. (2011). Callosal tracts and patterns of hemispheric dominance: A combined fMRI and DTI study. *NeuroImage, 54*, 779-786.

Hausmann, M., Kirk, I.J., and Corballis, M.C. (2004). Influence of task complexity on manual asymmetries. *Cortex, 40*, 103-110.

Karnath, H-O., Milner, D., and Vallar, G. (Eds.). (2002). *The Cognitive and Neural Basis of Spatial Neglect.* Oxford, UK and NY: Oxford University Press.

Keane, A.M. (1999). Cerebral organization of motor programming and verbal processing as a function of degree of hand preference and familial sinistrality. *Brain and Cognition*, *40*, 500-515.

Koeneke, S., Lutz, K., Essln, M., and Jancke, L. (2006). How finger tapping practice enhances efficiency of motor control. *NeuroReport, 17*, 1565-1569.

Lutz, K., Koeneke, S., Wustenberg, T., and Jancke, L. (2005). Asymmetry of cortical activation during maximum and convenient tapping speed. *Neuroscience Letters*, *373*, 61-66.

Lux, S., Keller, S., Mackay, C., Ebers, G., Marshall, J.C., Cherkas, L., Rezaie, R., Roberts, N., Fink, G.R., and Gurd, J.M. (2008). Crossed cerebral lateralization for verbal and visuo-spatial function in a pair of handedness discordant monozygotic twins: MRI and fMRI brain imaging. *Journal of Anatomy*, *212*, 235-248.

Marshall, J.C., and Fink, G. R. (2003). Cerebral localization, then and now. *NeuroImage, 20,* S2-S7.

Nalcaçi, E., Kalaycioglu, M., Cicek, M., and Genc, Y. (2001). The relationship between handedness and fine motor performance. *Cortex, 37,* 493 - 500.

Oldfield, R.C. (1971). The assessment and analysis of handedness: The Edinburgh Inventory. *Neuropsychologia, 9,* 97-113.

Passingham, R.E. and Toni, I. (2001). Contrasting the dorsal and ventral visual systems: Guidance of movement versus decision making. *NeuroImage, 14,* S125-S131.

Pisella, L., Gréa, H., Tilikete, C., Vighetto, A., Desmurget, M., Rode, G., Boisson, D., and Rossetti, Y. (2000). An 'automatic pilot' for the hand in human posterior parietal cortex: toward reinterpreting optic ataxia. *Nature Neuroscience, 3,* 729-736.

Pollock, B., Gross, J., and Schnitzler, A. (2006). Asymmetry of interhemispheric interaction in left-handed subjects. *Experimental Brain Research, 175,* 268-275.

Pollock, B., Rothkegel, H., Schnitzler, A., Paulus, W., and Lang, N. (2008). The effect of rTMS over left and right dorsolateral premotor cortex on movement timing of either hand. *European Journal Neuroscience, 27,* 757-764.

Ramnani, N. (2006). The primate cortico-cerebellar system: anatomy and function. *Nature Review Neuroscience, 7,* 511-522.

Rogalsky, C., Matchin, W., and Hickok, G. (2008). Broca's area, sentence Comprehension, and working memory: an fMRI study. *Frontiers in Human Neuroscience*, *2,* 14-27.

Rosch R.E., Ronan L., Cherkas L., and Gurd J. (2010a). Cerebellar asymmetry in a pair of monozygotic handedness discordant twins. *Journal of Anatomy*, *217*, 38-47.

Rosch R.E., Banissy M., Cherkas L., and Gurd J. (2010b). Hemispheric laterality discordance in several laterality measures for a pair of monozygotic handedness discordant twins. *Society for Neuroscience 2010*, San Diego CA Poster No. 912.7.

Rushworth, M.F.S., Johansen-Berg, H., Göbel, S.M., and Devlin, J.T. (2003). The left parietal and premotor cortices: motor attention and selection. *NeuroImage, 20*, S89-S100.

Serrien, D.J., Cassidy, J.M., and Brown, P. (2003). The importance of the dominant hemisphere in the organization of bimanual movements. *Human Brain Mapping, 18*, 296-305.

Serrien, D.J. (2008). Coordination constraints during bimanual versus unimanual performance conditions. *Neuropsychologia, 46*, 419-425.

Shulman, G.L., Pope, D.L.W., Astafiev, S.V., McAvoy, M. P., Snyder, A.Z., and Corbetta, M. (2010). Right hemisphere dominance during spatial selective attention and target detection occurs outside the dorsal fronto-parietal network. *Journal of Neuroscience, 30*, 3640-3651.

Stephan, K.E., Fink, G.R., and Marshall, J.C. (2007). Mechanisms of hemispheric specialization: insights from analyses of connectivity. *Neuropsychologia, 45*, 209-228.

Tapley, S.M., and Bryden, M.P. (1985). A group test for the assessment of performance between the hands. *Neuropsychologia, 23*, 289-304.

Verstynen, T., Diedrichsen, J., Albert, N., Aparico, P., and Ivry, R.B. (2005). Ipsilalteral motor cortex activity during unimanual hand movements relates to task complexity. *Journal of Neurophysiology, 93*, 1209-1222.

Witt, S.T., Meyerand, M.E., and Laird, A.R. (2008). Functional neuroimaging correlates of finger tapping task variations: An ALE meta-analysis. *NeuroImage, 42*, 343-356.

Yamomoto, S., and Kitazawa, S. (2001). Reversal of subjective temporal order due to arm crossing. *Nature Neuroscience, 4*, 759-765.

Yoon , U., Fahim, C., Perusse, D., and Evans, A.C. (2010). Lateralized genetic and environmental influences on human brain morphology of 8-year-old twins. *NeuroImage, 53*, 1117-1125.

Reviewed by Dr. P. Cowell, University of Sheffield, UK.

In: Handedness: Theories, Genetics and Psychology ISBN: 978-1-61470-502-4
Editors: J. Dunham and T. Davenport

Chapter VI

Electrostimulation Mapping and Language Lateralization in the Right Hemisphere

Vincent Lubrano[1,2] *and Franck-Emmanuel Roux*[1,2,*]
[1]UMR Unité 825, Université Paul Sabatier
Service de Neurochirurgie, Pole des Neurosciences,
[2]Centres Hospitalo-Universitaires, Toulouse, France

Abstract

Marc Dax is thought to have been the first to propose the doctrine of cerebral dominance, a model in which the faculty of language is controlled by the cerebral hemisphere contralateral to the preferred hand. Then, Broca and Wernicke described left hemispheric language dominance based on their anatomo- pathological findings in patients who presented clinically with aphasic disturbances. Since the 19th century, handedness has been associated with language dominance, though "Broca's rule" has been challenged by clinical and functional imaging studies, no latter than soon after its

* Corresponding author: Franck-Emmanuel Roux, Service de Neurochirurgie et INSERM 825, Hôpital Purpan, F-31059 Toulouse, France. Fax: +33 5 61 77 76 78. Tel: +33 6 10 42 04 28. E-mail: franck_emmanuel.roux@yahoo.fr

emergence and the brain representation of language in the right hemisphere still remains controversial.

To evaluate the role of handedness in language lateralization, we investigated 50 patients harboring right-sided brain tumors. There were 17 left-handers (33%) 33 right-handers (66%), who ranged in age from 22 to 78 years (mean: 50.4 years). These patients were all operated on using awake craniotomy procedures (i.e., their language was intraoperatively mapped by electrostimulation mapping prior to tumor resection).

Overall, 814 of 824 cortical sites (98.8%) were not associated with stimulation induced language deficit (Pre- and post-central gyri sensori-motor sites inferring with articulatory process of language were excluded from the analysis). Nevertheless, 8 of the 50 patients (16%) had at least one site where stimulation disrupted language function. We found that 4 out of 17 left-handers (23.5%) had positive language maps in their dominant hemisphere, whereas 4 out of 33 right-handers (12.2%) had positive language maps in their non-dominant hemisphere.

This stimulation mapping series is the largest ever-published one on the right hemisphere language mapping. Electrostimulation can detect non-motor language sites in the right hemisphere of left- but also right-handed patients although this is rare. Further exploratory studies are needed in the future to evaluate the clinical significance of RH naming sites and the possible aetiologies of the "atypical" localization of these language sites. Once, awake surgery could be useful to detect and spare language areas in some patients when surgery is considered in right hemisphere.

Keywords: Handedness, language right hemisphere, right hemisphere dominance, aphasia right hemisphere, stimulation mapping, brain tumors

Abbreviations

RH:	right hemisphere;
LH:	left hemisphere;
ESM:	electrostimulation mapping;
IAP:	intracarotid sodium amobarbital procedure;
fMRI:	functional magnetic resonance imaging.

Introduction

Marc Dax (1836) is thought to have been the first to propose the doctrine of cerebral dominance, a model in which the faculty of language is controlled by the cerebral hemisphere contralateral to the preferred hand. Then, *Broca (1861, 1863)* and *Wernicke (1874)* described left hemispheric language dominance based on their anatomo-pathological findings in patients who presented clinically with aphasic disturbances. Nevertheless, soon after the emergence of this theory, *John Hughlings Jackson (1868)* reported the first case of a left-handed man with a lesion of the right hemisphere and aphasia. He raised the possibility that language functions may be represented in both hemispheres. As Broca himself considered that not all patients have left hemispheric specialization for language, he defined the concept of an association between the dominant hand and the dominant hemisphere for language. According to this concept, the left hemisphere would be in charge of language in right-handers, whereas the right hemisphere would be dominant for left-handers. First exception of an intrinsic correlation between cerebral dominance for language and handedness came from *Byron Bramwell (1899)*, who introduced the concept of crossed-aphasia reporting the case a left-handed male exhibiting expressive aphasia after a lesion of the left hemisphere.

Since the 19th century, handedness has been associated with language dominance, though "Broca's rule" has been challenged by clinical studies (*Piercy 1960, Hécaen and Sauguet 1971, Luria 1976, Gloning 1977, Kimura 1983, Basso 1990*) showing that the relationship between manual preference and hemispheric dominance for language is far more complex. For example, Hécaen claimed that lesions of the right hemisphere result in aphasia in left-handers only, while left-hemisphere lesions had the same effects on language functions in left- and right-handers, albeit with more frequent troubles in comprehension in right-handers (*Hécaen and Sauguet 1971*) and spatial disorientation in left-handers (*Piercy 1960*). What emerged is that, more than 90% of right-handers and only 70% of left-handers, at most, show left hemisphere specialization for language (*Rasmussen 1977, Satz 1979*), and that variability is more important in left-handers, who are far more likely (30%) than right-handers (5%) to have speech controlled by the right hemisphere (*Hécaen and Sauguet 1971, Hécaen 1981*).

Language lateralization plays a major role in the decision-making and planning for supratentorial surgery of brain tumors. Since *Ojemann et al. (1989)* demonstrated that there was a great deal of language variability within the left hemisphere of adults with left lateralization of language, awake craniotomy with electrostimulation mapping (ESM) has become standard to map language function prior to surgical resection. However, this technique is based on the concept of this absence of right-hemisphere lateralization of language, and authors focused on the investigations in the left hemisphere (*Ojemann 1989, Roux 2003, Bello 2007, Sanai 2008, Duffau 2008a*). Hence, although considerable data has been accumulated on human language organization in the left dominant hemisphere, the brain representation of language in the right hemisphere remains controversial.

Notwithstanding, awake craniotomy with stimulation mapping also proved to be safe, practical and effective when routinely and/or non-selectively used for tumors implicating left or right hemispheres (*Serletis 2007, Sacko 2011*). To evaluate the impact of handedness on the degree of language lateralization, we investigated 50 patients harboring brain tumors involving their right hemisphere, which were operated on using awake craniotomy procedures.

Methods

Patients

From 2002 to 2007, 50 patients with brain tumors were consecutively subjected to awake craniotomy for resective surgery in their right hemisphere. Patients' population characteristics are summarized in Table 1. There were 28 males (56%) and 22 females (44%) who ranged in age from 22 to 78 years (mean: 50.4 years). No patients had symptoms of raised intracranial pressure or intractable epilepsy. All the patients included in this study underwent volumetric baseline and post contrast MR imaging scans before surgery. All the patients and their families gave their informed consent to study their language areas by direct brain mapping. All data related to the patients' surgery were prospectively entered into a database immediately after surgery. Histology was classified according to the World Health Organization brain tumor classification.

Pre- and Postoperative Assessments

The pre- and postoperative assessments were done within 10 days before the surgery and during the postoperative course, within 10 days after surgery and at 2-3 months after.

Table 1. Population characteristics

Patient population characteristics (n=50)	
Age – years	
Median	50.4
Range	22 - 78
Sex – no. (%)	
Male	28 (56%)
Female	22 (44%)
Signs and symptoms at presentation – no. (%)	
Seizure	25 (50%)
Hemiparesis	10 (20%)
Paresthesia	4 (8%)
Anomic symptoms	0 (0%)
Headache	4 (8%)
Cognitive deficit	4 (8%)
Confusion	2 (4%)
None	5 (10%)
Tumor type	
Glioma	
WHO Grade 2	14
WHO Grade 3	6
Glioblastoma	14
Meningioma	3
Cavernoma	3
Brain Metastasis	9
Other	1

Table 2. Handedness scores in our population

Handedness by the Edinburgh Inventory	
Right-handers – *no. (%)*	33 (67%)
Mean score (range)	88 (60; 100)
Left-handers – *no. (%)*	17 (33%)
Mean score (range)	-44 (-100; -10)

All patients had general and neurological clinical examination. We assessed handedness by submitting the patients to the Edinburgh Inventory Questionnaire (*Oldfield 1971*). Language testing was conducted by the neurological and neurosurgical team, who evaluated oral understanding, naming, and oral fluency by using appropriate tests. Preoperatively, no dysphasic patient whose errors went up by more than 10% in this testing was included in the study. Postoperatively, language assessments were conducted to demonstrate whether surgery resulted in stability, improvement or deterioration of language functions.

Stimulation Mapping

The patients were all operated on during an awake craniotomy. In our institution, it is used either to map sensorimotor cortex in addition to language cortex (i.e. mostly in case of central tumors). The brain was exposed in a standard fashion. We used a neuronavigation system (Medtronic, Tolochenaz, Switzerland) to localize the tumor and guide the mapping procedure in all patients.

Intraoperative cortical stimulation was used to localize functional cortex after determination of the afterdischarge threshold by electrocorticography. The cortex was directly stimulated, using the bipolar electrode of the NIMBUS® Multi-functional Stimulator (1mm electrodes separated by 5mm – Newmedic®, Toulouse, France). The current amplitude was progressively increased by .5mA, beginning at 2mA. We used biphasic square-wave pulses of 1ms at 60Hz, with maximum train duration of 4sec. Slides of black and white drawings of common objects were presented to the patient, who performed overt object naming from object images. Speech arrest, anomia, semantic and phonological paraphasia, circumlocution were scored as errors.

Electrical stimulation in the primary sensorimotor area of the face can disrupt speech because of an inability to move the tongue, the eyes, or other distal muscles of the face or extremities. These 'motor effect areas' (*Luders 2007*) were excluded from analysis in this study. To be accepted as positive sites, each language error sites we found was meticulously tested 3 times. Those sites showing no reproducible language errors were not included. A sterile ticket of .25cm2 marked each positive site we found. Intraoperative photographs of the brain showing the positive cortical stimulation sites were taken. Mapping procedures were video-recorded as evidence of each patient's cortical organization and so that the patient's responses could be further analyzed in team meetings. After each case analysis, the site of speech production error was prospectively entered into an excel sheet database.

Results

Handedness

Our brain-tumor-patient population included 17 left-handers (34%) and 33 right-handers (66%). Their handedness scores (Edinburgh Inventory Questionnaire) are summarized in Table 2. They were distributed as follows: the mean score in right-handers was 88.0 (range: 60; 100) and the mean score in left-handers was -44.4 (range: -100; -10).

Stimulation Maps

Cortical localization of language areas was undertaken in all patients with no difficulties. Current intensity necessary for language mapping ranged from 4.3mA to 7.5mA. No patient had intraoperative generalized seizure.

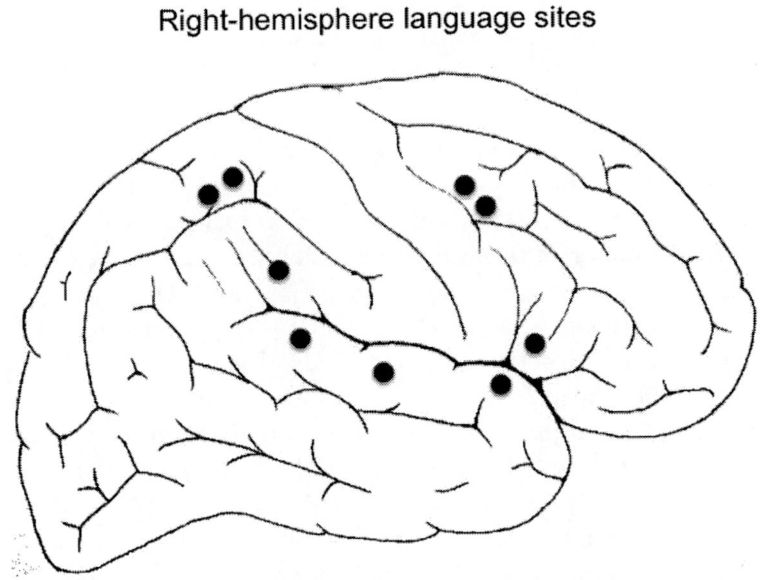

Figure 1. Schematic illustration of the localization of positive language mapping sites (•). Two sites were found in the middle frontal gyrus, 1 in the inferior frontal gyrus, 3 in the superior temporal gyrus, 1 in the supramarginal gyrus, and 2 sites were detected in the superior parietal lobe.

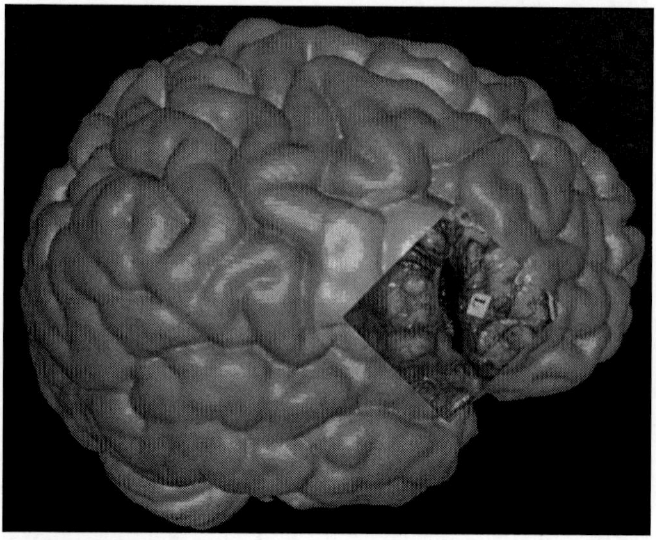

Figure 2. Illustrative case. 3D right lateral view of the brain of a 44-year-old left-handed (-50% according to the *Edinburgh* Inventory) man harboring an infiltrative WHO-grade-II astrocytoma. No language deficit was revealed preoperatively after language testing. Awake fronto-temporal craniotomy was performed. Superimposed post-resection intraoperative photograph shows one positive (L) essential language site (speech arrest) that has been found in the right opercular cortex.

Cumulatively, 824 cortical sites were stimulated among all patients. The composite map of all positive language sites we elicited by ESM is shown in Figure 1. These interference sites were localized in small cortical areas (< 1 cm2) and distributed in the right hemisphere as follows: 3 sites in the frontal lobe, 3 sites in the temporal lobe and 3 sites in the parietal lobe. Overall, 9 naming sites were detected in 8 patients, whereas no naming site was detected in 42 patients. Five language sites were detected in 4 left-handers, while four language sites were detected in 4 right-handers.

The types of language errors induced by stimulation mapping according to their localization are shown in Table 3. All but one site generating speech arrest were localized in the posterior part of the Broca area in the pars opercularis (BA44/6) (see illustrative case in Figure 2) or the posterior part of the midfrontal gyrus in the premotor cortex (BA 9/6). Anomia, semantic paraphasia, and hesitations were observed in the superior temporal gyrus (BA38, BA22 and Wernicke area). Speech arrest was also noted in the supramarginal gyrus (BA40) and hesitations in the upper parietal lobe (BA7). No phonemic paraphasia was found.

Relationship between Handedness and Stimulation Maps

We found that 13 out of 17 left-handers (76%) had negative language maps in their right hemisphere, whereas 4 out of 33 right-handers (12%) had positive language maps in their right hemisphere. The relationship between the degree of handedness by the Edinburgh Inventory and the occurrence of language disruption when stimulating the right hemisphere by ESM is stressed in Table 4. Globally, the more left-handed the patients were, the higher was the occurrence of language disruption when applying stimulation mapping on the right hemisphere cortex, and vice versa (p=0.521, *Fisher test*).

Postoperative Assessments

As compared to the baseline preoperative assessment, 6 patients experienced a transient new motor deficit, which resolved in the days after surgery, whereas one patient who had a severe hemiparesis significantly improved. One patient had aphasic troubles in addition to dysarthria associated with brachio-facial paresis. These symptoms almost completely disappeared in the weeks after surgery.

Table 3. Types and localizations of language errors

	Language errors induced by stimulation mapping according to their localization			
	speech arrest	anomia	semantic paraphasia	hesitations
Op. IFG	1			
Post. MFG	2			
Ant. STG			1	
Mid. STG		1		
Post. STG				1
Ant. SMG	1			
Sup. PL				2

Op. IFG: Inferior Frontal Gyrus, *pars opercularis* ; Post. MFG: posterior part of the Mid-Frontal Gyrus; Ant., Mid., Post. STG: respectively anterior, middle and posterior parts of the Superior Temporal Gyrus; Ant. SMG: anterior part of the SupraMarginal Gyrus; Sup. PL : Superior Parietal Lobule.

Table 4. Relationship between the degree of handedness by the Edinburgh Inventory and the occurrence of language disruption when stimulating the right hemisphere by ESM (p=0.521, *Fisher test*)

Handedness	-99 or less	More than -99; -75 or less	More than -75; -25 or less	More than -25; 25 or less	More than 25; 75 or less	More than 75; 99 or less	More than 99
Number of patients - n	1	2	10	4	4	19	10
At least one positive stimulation mapping site within the right hemisphere – n (*%)*	0 (0%)	0 (0%)	3 (30%)	1 (25%)	1 (25%)	3 (16%)	0 (0%)

Discussion

The main findings of this study may be summarized as follows: i) the degree of handedness seems related in a nonrandom fashion to the risk of language disruption when mapping the right hemisphere; ii) language cortex can be detected by direct cortical stimulation in the right hemisphere of left-handers as well as right-handers (based on Edinburgh Inventory test) even in the "nondominant" hemisphere.

Handedness, Functional Imaging, and Language Lateralization

Various methods have been developed to assess the laterality of language production in a valid and more or less invasive way. Intracarotid sodium amobarbital procedure (IAP) was introduced in 1949 by Wada, who noted that the intracarotid injection of amobarbital performed in an attempt to investigate inter-hemispheric spread of epileptiform discharges produced a transient ipsilateral paralysis of hemispheric function without eliciting unacceptable sedation or interruption of vital functions (*Wada 1960*). This technique became standard to determine hemispheric language dominance. IAP was used by *Rasmussen and Milner (1975)*, who reported that whereas 95% of right-handers have articulate language lateralized to the LH, only 70% of left-handers have similar organization, with 15% having RH and 15% bilateral representation. More recent functional imaging studies (*Pujol 1999, Knecht 2000, Szaflarski 2002*) estimated the prevalence of complete right hemisphere dominance in healthy left-handed individuals is estimated to be up to 22% and in right-handed individuals as high as 7.5%. Combining functional Doppler ultrasonography (fTCD) and functional magnetic resonance imaging (fMRI), *Knecht et al. (2000)* provided evidence that 4% of a randomly selected sample of strong right-handers were RH-dominant for language production, against 27% of the strong left-handers. Moreover, it has also been stressed in this study that there is a graded continuum from left hemispheric to right hemispheric language lateralization in healthy subjects. Language lateralization proved to be not necessarily dichotomous, and *Knecht et al. (2000)* advocated a consistent and almost linear relationship between the degree of handedness and the direction of language dominance.

We found quite similar results as overall the number of patients having positive language map decreased while their handedness scores increased. However, our sample of strong left-handed patients (handedness $\leq$ -75, n=3) was too small to be analyzed, and further data will be necessary before drawing a definitive conclusion.

Handedness and Stimulation Mapping Studies of the Right Hemisphere

Few stimulation mapping studies reported language investigations conducted prior to right hemisphere surgery in the context of right hemispheric dominance or bilateral representation of language. *Duffau et al. (2008b)* documented the cortico-subcortical organization of language in the RH of nine left-handers. In their population, the Edinburgh test scores ranged from −70 to −100. Interestingly, five patients had preoperative partial seizures with transient language disturbances, and all the nine patients presented transient language disorders in the immediate postoperative period. Their results provided strong arguments in favor of a language distribution pattern quite similar to the one classically reported in the LH in right-handers (*Ojemann 1989, Duffau 2008a*). *Chang et al. (2010),* studying the organization of essential language sites in the right hemisphere of 15 patients (10 left-handers, 4 ambidextrous, and one right-hander whom experienced significant preoperative language deficit) reported similar cortical results. Consistent with *Ojemann et al. (1989)*, considerable variability was observed between patients with respect to location of essential cortical language sites in this latter study.

Reports describing language mapping in exclusive RH dominance in purely right-handed patients are even scarce. *Oishi et al. (2006)* reported a patient with a right frontal tumor, who was strongly right-handed but had aphasic seizures and was dominant for speech on the right hemisphere by Wada test. Using subdural electrodes, they observed that stimulation over the right inferior frontal gyrus disrupted counting, spontaneous speech, and object naming. They concluded they found Broca area, in a case of provoked crossed aphasia (i.e. right-hemisphere transient lesion in this right-handed individual). *Vassal et al. (2010)* also identified cortical language areas (in the frontal and temporal lobes) and white matter language pathways in three strongly right-handed patients with right-sided tumors, which again favors the hypothesis of a mirror organization between the RH and the LH.

Our data are globally concordant with these aforementioned results: pattern of language sites distribution in the hemisphere and their associated error-types is similar for the right and the left hemisphere provided that the considered hemisphere is "dominant" or the language bilaterally organized.

Stimulation Mapping Studies of the Right "Nondominant" Hemisphere

Language function was rarely evaluated in the right non-dominant hemisphere using stimulation mapping. *Bhatnagar and Andy (1983)* explored the right cortex of 3 patients undergoing cortical resection for intractable seizures. Despite negative Wada's test, ESM impaired linguistic function when applied in their right nondominant hemisphere. Tasks they used were of increasing complexity (from object naming to responsive naming). They speculated a right nondominant language system anatomically and functionally tied to the left dominant one. This system would be passively involved, its integrity not being "essential" to language production under normal conditions. Interestingly, *Jabbour et al. (2005)*, who were the first to publish ESM of language areas in the right hemisphere in epilepsy patients with bilateral language representation on Wada testing, identified language cortex, which they named "accessory language areas in relation to the LH".

Such hypothesis matches well with clinical observations showing contribution of the RH to word production in right-handers (*Joanette 1988*). Furthermore and contrary to early notions that articulation generation was solely a function of the LH, functional imaging research makes it increasingly apparent that both hemispheres are involved in the production of expressive language (*Riecker 2002, Ackermann and Riecker 2004, Kemeny 2005*). The RH has been shown to supplement the LH, which is crucially responsible for the programming of motor commands necessary for speech production, by controlling the prosodic and nonpropositional components of expressive language (*Buchanan 2000, Alho 2003, Shibata 2007*).

Our data supports the implication of the nondominant RH in language, as language sites have been found in the right hemisphere of right-handers, who have not been selected because of RH dominance on IAP, fMRI, or preoperative aphasic symptoms as in previous studies (*Duffau 2010b, Chang 2010*). This is probably the reason why the rate of negative site in our study is very high (98.8%) as compared to the one (83.7%) of *Chang et al. (2010)*.

Furthermore, since the language areas we found in the subgroup of 4 right-handers were located in the vicinity (≤2cm) of the rolandic cortex and half of them generated speech arrest, one could have hypothesized they may correspond to a reorganization of the sensorimotor cortex (*Duffau 2003*). However, two arguments can be opposed to such alternative view: (1) 'motor effect' areas were ruled out by carefully checking inability to move the tongue, the eyes, or other distal muscles of the face or extremities that may have been associated with inability to speak; (2) since the 4 right-handers exhibited various types of tumors including noninfiltrative lesions as metastasis and cavernoma (eg, as opposed to infiltrative gliomas), interindividual variability and mass effect were more likely to explain this distribution than brain plasticity (*Lubrano 2010*).

Limitations

Before concluding, several methodological limitations of our study have to be stressed. First, our population was unselected. Then though it is representative of the right-sided brain tumor patients' population, it included few strongly left-handers, which limited data analyze in the relation to this subgroup. Second, as our primary goal was to determine the impact of handedness on language lateralization as assessed by ESM, our population was not preoperatively investigated by functional investigations such as IAP or fMRI. It would be interesting in the future to combine these preoperative investigations to ESM and compare their results. Third, the exposure of the cortex is necessary limited to the boundaries of the lesion in the context of brain-tumor surgery, and language cortex may be found distant to this region because of native language organization or postlesional reorganization, especially in slow-growing lesions (*Desmurget 2007*).

Conclusion

In this series, which to the best of our knowledge is the largest ever published, ESM elicited naming language sites in the right hemisphere of left- and right-handers exhibiting various scores of handedness. Our data plead for a graded continuum from left hemispheric to right hemispheric language lateralization. Electrostimulation can detect non-motor language sites in the right hemisphere of left- but also right-handed patients although this is rare. Further exploratory studies are needed in the future to evaluate the clinical significance of RH naming sites and the possible aetiologies of the "atypical" localization of these language sites. Once, awake surgery could be useful to detect and spare language areas in some patients when surgery is considered in right hemisphere.

References

Ackermann, H., and Riecker, A. (2004). The contribution of the insula to motor aspects of speech production: A review and a hypothesis. *Brain and Language,* 89, 320–328.

Alho K, Vorobyev VA, Medvedev SV, Pakhomov SV, Roudas MS, Tervaniemi M, et al: Hemispheric lateralization of cerebral blood-flow changes during selective listening to dichotically presented continuous speech. *Brain Res Cogn Brain* Res 17:201–211, 2003.

Basso A, Farabola M, Grassi MP, Laiacona M, Zanobio ME. Aphasia in left-handers. Comparison of aphasia profiles and language recovery in non-right-handed and matched right-handed patients. *Brain Lang.* 1990 Feb;38(2):233-52.

Bello L, Gallucci M, Fava M, Carrabba G, Giussani C, Acerbi F, Baratta P, Songa V, Conte V, Branca V, Stocchetti N, Papagno C, Gaini SM. Intraoperative subcortical language tract mapping guides surgical removal of gliomas involving speech areas. *Neurosurgery.* 2007 Jan;60(1):67-80; discussion 80-2.

Bhatnagar S, Andy OJ. Language in the nondominant right hemisphere. *Arch Neurol.* 1983 Nov;40(12):728-31.

Buchanan TW, Lutz K, Mirzazade S, Specht K, Shah NJ, Zilles K, et al: Recognition of emotional prosody and verbal components of spoken language: an fMRI study. *Brain Res Cogn Brain Res* 9:227–238, 2000.

Bramwell, B. (1899). On ''crossed'' aphasia. *Lancet* (June 3), 1473–1479.

Broca P. Nouvelle observation d'aphémie par une lésion de la moitié postérieure des deuxième et troisième circonvolution frontales gauches. *Bull Soc Anat* 1861;36:398-407.

Broca P. Localisations des fonctions cérébrales: siège de la faculté du langage articulé. *Bull. Soc. Anthropol.* 1863;4:200-8.

Chang EF, Wang DD, Perry DW, Barbaro NM, Berger MS. Homotopic organization of essential language sites in right and bilateral cerebral hemispheric dominance. *J Neurosurg.* 2011 Apr;114(4):893-902.

Desmurget M, Bonnetblanc F, Duffau H. Contrasting acute and slow-growing lesions: a new door to brain plasticity. *Brain.* 2007 Apr;130(Pt 4):898-914.

Duffau H, Capelle L, Denvil D, Sichez N, Gatignol P, Lopes M, Mitchell MC, Sichez JP, Van Effenterre R. Functional recovery after surgical resection of low grade gliomas in eloquent brain: hypothesis of brain compensation. *J Neurol Neurosurg Psychiatry.* 2003 Jul;74(7):901-7.

Duffau H, Peggy Gatignol ST, Mandonnet E, Capelle L, Taillandier L. Intraoperative subcortical stimulation mapping of language pathways in a consecutive series of 115 patients with Grade II glioma in the left dominant hemisphere. *J Neurosurg.* 2008 Sep;109(3):461-71.

Duffau H, Leroy M, Gatignol P. Cortico-subcortical organization of language networks in the right hemisphere: an electrostimulation study in left-handers. *Neuropsychologia.* 2008 Dec;46(14):3197-209.

Gloning K. Handedness and aphasia. *Neuropsychologia* 1977; 15: 355–8.

Hécaen H, Sauguet J. Cerebral dominance in left-handed subjects. *Cortex.* 1971 Mar;7(1):19-48.

Hécaen H, De Agostini M, Monzon-Montes A. Cerebral organization in left-handers. *Brain Lang.* 1981 Mar;12(2):261-84.

Jabbour RA, Hempel A, Gates JR, Zhang W, Risse GL. Right hemisphere language mapping in patients with bilateral language. *Epilepsy Behav.* 2005 Jun;6(4):587-92.

Jackson J: Deficit of intellectual expression (aphasia) with left hemiplegia. *Lancet* 1:457, 1868 (Letter).

Joanette Y, Goulet P, Le Dorze G. Impaired word naming in right-brain-damaged right-handers: error types and time-course analyses. *Brain Lang.* 1988 May;34(1):54-64.

Kemeny S, Ye FQ, Birn R, Braun AR. Comparison of continuous overt speech fMRI using BOLD and arterial spin labeling. *Hum Brain Mapp.* 2005 Mar;24(3):173-83.

Kimura D, Speech representation in an unbiased sample of left-handers. *Human Ncurobiol* (1983) 2: 147 -1 S4.

Knecht S, Dräger B, Deppe M, Bobe L, Lohmann H, Flöel A, Ringelstein EB, Henningsen H. Handedness and hemispheric language dominance in healthy humans. *Brain.* 2000 Dec;123 Pt 12:2512-8.

Lubrano V, Draper L, Roux FE. What makes surgical tumor resection feasible in Broca's area? Insights into intraoperative brain mapping. *Neurosurgery.* 2010 May;66(5):868-75

Luria AR. *Basic problems in neurolinguistics.* The Hague: Mouton ; 1976.

Lüders HO. Crossed aphasia elicited by direct cortical stimulation. *Neurology.* 2007 May 8;68(19):1638-9

Oishi M, Suzuki K, Sasaki O, Nakazato S, Kitazawa K, Takao T, Koike T. Crossed aphasia elicited by direct cortical stimulation. *Neurology.* 2006 Oct 10;67(7):1306-7.

Ojemann G, Ojemann J, Lettich E, Berger M. Cortical language localization in left, dominant hemisphere. An electrical stimulation mapping investigation in 117 patients. *J Neurosurg. 1989* Sep;71(3):316-26.

Oldfield RC. The assessment and analysis of handedness: the Edinburgh inventory. *Neuropsychologia* 1971 ; 9 :97-113

Piercy M, Hecaen H, de Ajuriaguerra. Constructional apraxia associated with unilateral cerebral lesions-left and right sided cases compared. *Brain.* 1960;83:225-42.

Pujol J, Deus J, Losilla JM, Capdevila A. Cerebral lateralization of language in normal left-handed people studied by functional MRI. *Neurology.* 1999 Mar 23;52(5):1038-43.

Rasmussen T, Milner B. The role of early left-brain injury in determining lateralization of cerebral speech functions. *Annals of the New York Academy of Science,* 1977, 299: 355-369.

Riecker A, Wildgruber D, Dogil G, Grodd W, Ackermann H. Hemispheric lateralization effects of rhythm implementation during syllable repetitions: an fMRI study. *Neuroimage.* 2002 May;16(1):169-76.

Roux FE, Boulanouar K, Lotterie JA, Mejdoubi M, LeSage JP, Berry I. Language functional magnetic resonance imaging in preoperative assessment of language areas: correlation with direct cortical stimulation. *Neurosurgery.* 2003 Jun;52(6):1335-45; discussion 1345-7.

Sacko O, Lauwers-Cances V, Brauge D, Sesay M, Brenner A, Roux FE. Awake craniotomy versus surgery under general anesthesia for resection of supratentorial lesions. *Neurosurgery.* 2011 Jan 26.

Sanai N, Mirzadeh Z, Berger MS. Functional outcome after language mapping for glioma resection. *N Engl J Med.* 2008 Jan 3;358(1):18-27.

Satz, P. (1979). A test of somemodels of hemispheric speech organization in the left and right-handed. *Science,* 203, 1131–1133.

Serletis D, Bernstein M. Prospective study of awake craniotomy used routinely and nonselectively for supratentorial tumors. *J Neurosurg.* 2007 Jul;107(1):1-6.

Shibata M, Abc J, Terao A, Miyamoto T. Neural mechanisms involved in the comprehension of metaphoric and literal sentences: an fMRI study. *Brain Res.* 2007 Aug 29;1166:92-102.

Szaflarski JP, Binder JR, Possing ET, McKiernan KA, Ward BD, Hammeke TA: Language lateralization in left-handed and ambidextrous people: fMRI data. *Neurology* 59:238–244, 2002.

Vassal M, Le Bars E, Moritz-Gasser S, Menjot N, Duffau H. Crossed aphasia elicited by intraoperative cortical and subcortical stimulation in awake patients. *J Neurosurg.* 2010 Dec;113(6):1251-8.

Wada J, Rasmussen T (1960) Intracarotid injection of sodiurn amy tal for the latcralization of cerebral speech dominance: experimental and clinical observations. *J Neurosurg* 17:266-282, 1960.

Wernicke C. *Der aphasische Symptomenkomplex: Eine psychologische Studie auf anatomischer Basis.* Breslau: Max Cohn and Wegert; 1874.

In: Handedness: Theories, Genetics and Psychology ISBN: 978-1-61470-502-4
Editors: J. Dunham and T. Davenport

Chapter VII

Handedness, Achievement in Sport and Boxing*

Recep Gursoy[1], Mehmet Akif Ziyagil[2], Suleyman Sahin[3], and Senol Dane[4]

[1]Ataturk University, Department of Physical Education and Sport, Erzurum, Turkey

[2]Amasya University, Department of Physical Education and Sport, Amasya, Turkey

[3]Yildirim Manucipality, Department of Sport Education, Bursa, Turkey

[4]Ataturk University, Medical Faculty, Department of Physiology, Erzurum, Turkey

Abstract

Handedness is a preference for the use of one of the right- or the left-hands. In the large majority of right-handers, speech is controlled by the left side of the brain. Also, the right hemisphere of the brain is usually specialized for recognizing and remembering faces and understanding

* A version of this chapter also appears in Advancements in the Scientific Study of Combative Sports, edited by Jason E. Warnick and W. Daniel Martin, published by Nova Science Publishers, Inc. It was submitted for appropriate modifications in an effort to encourage wider dissemination of research.

relationships in space. We live in a right-handed world and that left-handers have an inherent disadvantage in using tools designed for right-handers. Left-handed persons are believed to have better developed motor, attentional and spatial functions. Some studies have explored a possible correlation between left-handedness and enhanced performance in specific sports such as baseball, cricket, fencing, soccer and tennis. The rate of the left-handed boxers was higher compared to the right-handed ones in the National Road Sport Men Boxing Club in Turkey. These results may be associated with two suggestions: 1. the left-handed subjects have an intrinsic advantage over right-handers due to superior spatio-motor skills, 2. advantage in the left-handed boxer and the left-handed other athletes may result from the nature of the game (boxing) or frequency-dependent strategic advantage.

Handedness

Handedness is a preference for the use of one of the right- or the left-hands. Although many animals have a preferred paw or hand (50% for right and 50% for left), only humans have a typical preference for the right hand. Approximately equal incidence of left- and right-hand and paw preferences have been reported in mammals such as chimpanzees (Finch, 1941), rhesus monkey (Warren, 1953; Milner, 1969; Gautrin and Ettlinger, 1970), bonnet monkeys (Broker, Lehman, Heimbuch, and Kidd, 1981), cats (Cole, 1955), mice (Collins, 1969), and rats (Annett, 1985). Approximately 75 percent of the human population is strongly right-handed, and approximately 90 percent is predominantly right-handed. Among the remaining 10 percent, a great deal of variability exists. Some people are strongly left-handed, and others, called ambidextrous, are left-handed for some activities and right-handed for others.

Previc (1991) hypothesized that cerebral lateralization in humans derives from the asymmetric prenatal development of handedness, and by extension, of the ear and labyrinth (vestibular organ). According to this hypothesis, the aural asymmetry is a manifest advantage in monaural sensitivity of the right ear at birth, presumably derived from an enhanced middle-ear conduction caused by a smaller right embryonic craniofacial region. Dane and Bayirli (1998) reported that right-handers had a mean right ear advantage and left-handers had a mean left advantage by assessing durations of hearing for right and left ears in young healthy subjects. About two-thirds of humans possess a slightly larger left facial region (Burke, 1971; Vig and Hewitt, 1975) which is thought to originate during early fetal development (Trenouth, 1985). Keles at al. (1997) reported that facial areas on the left are significantly larger than those on the right in right-handers and that left-handers are inconsistent in facial asymmetry, but they tend to have larger facial areas on the right than on the left. Dane and Bayirli (1998) suggested that hand preference may be related to facial and aural sensitivity asymmetries. Dane et al. (2004) reported and suggested that handedness was associated with the left face width especially for women. The left facial region was larger for right-handers than left-handers. The smaller measure for the left face of left-handers might be associated with an advantage of left ear sensitivity.

Scientific studies conducted during the 1970s and early '80s suggest that differences in left- and right-handers in patterns of brain organization may be associated with differences in skills, aptitudes, and perhaps even personalities. In the large majority of right-handers, speech is controlled by the left side of the brain. The right hemisphere of the brain is usually specialized for recognizing and remembering faces and understanding relationships in space. In left-handers, the pattern of brain organization is unpredictable. About 65 to 70 percent of left-handers have speech controlled by the left hemisphere of the brain, as is the case for right-handers, but in 30 to 35 percent of left-handers speech is controlled by the right hemisphere. In some left-handers, both hemispheres of the brain are capable of controlling speech.

The hand an individual comes to prefer is determined, in part, by genetics, but this does not mean, for example, that two right-handed parents cannot have a left-handed child, or the reverse. The precise mechanisms by which genes affect handedness are still unknown. A physical injury may also be involved. During the birth process, the region of the brain controlling the hand is sometimes damaged, so that a child who would have been right-handed without such damage becomes left-handed.

Social pressures have had a considerable effect on handedness. In the United States and many other countries, using the left hand for writing was once strongly discouraged. Language records the negative views historically associated with left-handedness. The word *sinister*, meaning “evil,” also means “left-handed,” and the French word for “left,” *gauche*, is also commonly used to mean “awkward.” Left-handers are, of course, no more awkward than right-handers; any awkwardness or psychological disturbances observed in left-handers in the past could well be attributed to the problems that were created for them by an intolerant society. Many famous persons, including Leonardo da Vinci, Benjamin Franklin, and Lewis Carroll, were left-handed.

Handedness and Motor Abilities

It is often said that we live in a right-handed world and that left-handers have an inherent disadvantage in using tools designed for right-handers. When right and left-handers are compared on tasks in which levers or knobs have to be manipulated to control target displays, it is important to be sure that each handedness group has equal opportunity to move the controls in the preferred direction. For example, Bradley (1957) found right-handers more likely to turn knobs clockwise and to expect clockwise rotations to increase and counterclockwise relations to decrease the variable controlled; left-handers did not show a clear directional preference. On a motor task reported by Davis, Wehrkamp, and Smith (1951) on which right-handers were faster than left-handers, the manipulations were all clockwise, which might have given the right-handers an advantage.

Chapanis and Gropper (1968) compared 32 right-handers and 32 left-handers in setting dials where movements had to be made in either direction, by either hand, and when the relationship between direction of turn and changes in display were either in accord or discord with the usual expectation (clockwise movements associated with display changes from left to right or upward, and anticlockwise movements with from right to left or downward). The errors made by right- and left-handers using each hand varied considerably with the differing display control relationships. Over-all there was not much difference between right-and left-handers in using their preferred hand. However, left-handers were considerably better than right-handers in using their non-preferred hands. When the direction the direction of display control relationship was opposite to that generally expected, left-handers did relatively better than right-handers with both hands, and right-handers, did relatively better with their left hands than for he usual relationship). Annett and Sheridan (1973) also found that right-handers were better at using the left hand than the right hand when the display control relationship was reversed for moving a lever to control a visual display. Grant and Kaestner (1955) found that right-handers tracked right-to-left targets better than left-to-right targets and left-handers vice versa, but there was no over all difference between right-and left-handers in tracking with a hand-wheel control.

Two studies of speed of writing by right-and left-handed children found no significant differences (Reed and Smith, 1962; Smith and Reed 1959). Flowers (1975) compared right, left, and ambilateral handers (any mixture of preference fort he left and right hands) on two tasks, one of visually controlled aiming between handedness group for the non-preferred hand on aiming task and no difference for either hand on the tapping task. The one significant difference between groups was that ambilaterals were slower than task. Peters and Durding (1979) compared right- and left-handers for speed of tapping by each hand. The handedness groups were virtually identical fort he preferred hand, but left-handers were significantly faster than right-handers with their non-preferred hand.

Comparisons of right- and left-handers for hand control found no difference between groups for steadiness (Simon, 1964) or for capacity for independent finger movement by each hand (Parlow, 1978). Kimura and Vanderwolf (1970) found right-handers better than left-handers in task of independent finger movement in one experiment but did not confirm this difference in a second experiment.

In contrast to the above laboratory-based tasks, motor skills in sports performance can also be compared between handedness groups. Way (1958) asked whether women enrolled in college physical education programs differ in motor ability between groups classified as mixed or consistent for hand, eye, and foot preferences. She reported the mixed group superior for skill in archery, bowling, badminton, and tennis. Porac and Coren (1981) collected questionnaire data on the hand, eye, and foot preferences of 2611 athletes in a variety of sports. They found that athletes rated as in the top levels of proficiency differed from controls in being less consistently right-sided.

The analyses for particular sports must be interpreted cautiously as the numbers of respondents for each sport were not given. Further, when nine comparisons were made for each of 15 sports, some differences at the 5 % level of significance would be expected by chance, as Porac and Coren acknowledged. Comparisons for left-and right-sidedness of hand, foot, and eye found that the only advantage for a handedness group occurred for left-handed boxers. Advantages for eyedness were found to be left for basketball and gymnastics and right for bowling. Comparisons for mixed versus consistent preferences (for a questionnaire asking 4, 3, and 3 questions about hand, foot, or eye preference, respectively) and for crossed versus congruent preferences (for hand-foot, hand-eye and foot-eye) found other significant effects. Very few of these were in favor of consistent sidedness (mainly shooting and racquet sports), and the remainder favored not consistent sidedness (including baseball, basketball, soccer, field and ice hockey, and gymnastics).

Hand Preference and Hand Skill

The idea of hand preference implies some greater skill for the preferred hand. We say that a person is right handed if he uses his right hand rather than his left to carry out the more skilled kinds of movement and is more skilful at such movements with the right hand than with his left. The converse is true of a left handed person (Brain, 1945). It is currently fashionable to stress the weakness of the relationship between hand preference and hand skill (Porac and Coren, 1981). An evaluation of this judgment depends on questions about the nature of skill and whether psychologists have succeeded in measuring it, as well as questions about whether psychologists have been successful in measuring hand preference.

While attention is focused on hand preference alone, there are no independent criteria against which to judge the significance of particular patterns of preference. If hand preference could be systematically and reliably related to something else, then we would have an objective standard against which to evaluate preference data. This point is fundamental, in our view to the problem of analyzing handedness. It is analogous to the problem of how to define a point in space. This was not possible until the system of coordinates was invented. If hand preference can be coordinated with an independent measure of hand skill, then the elusive phenomenon can be regarded as pinned down.

Left-Handedness and Success in Sport

One neuro-developmental theory (Geschwind and Galaburda, 1985a, 1985b, 1987) posits that left-handed persons have a larger right-hemisphere than right-handed persons, due to varying levels of prenatal hormones and their effects on hemispheric development in utero. As a result, left-handed persons are believed to have better developed motor, attentional and spatial functions (Geschwind and Galaburda, 1985a, 1985b, 1987; Nass and Gazzaniga, 1987). To test this theory of brain development indirectly, researchers (e.g., McLean and Ciurczak, 1982; Bisiacchi, Ripoll, Stein, Simonet and Azemar, 1985; Wood and Aggleton, 1989; Grondin, Guiard, Ivry and Koren, 1999) have explored a possible correlation between left-handedness and enhanced performance in specific sports (viz., baseball, cricket, fencing, football [soccer], and tennis). One difficulty in interpreting the published findings is that for many of the sports examined, athletic performance is often the result of team effort, not solely due to individual performance. Fencing and singles tennis, however, are non-team sports; thus, they lend themselves particularly well to testing the hypothesis that left-handed competitors may have superior visuo-spatial and visuo-motor skill compared to their right-handed opponents.

Several studies have explored a possible left-handed advantage in professional tennis (Annett, 1985; Azemar, Ripoll, Simonet and Stein, 1983; Wood and Aggleton, 1989). The findings of these reports are equivocal, due to the shortcomings that they: (a) examined merely one tournament (Wimbledon); (b) combined data from amateur-only and professional-only tournaments; (c) largely focused on male players; (d) examined data within a limited time frame (e.g., one to three years); (e) often failed to compare observed rates of left handedness in tournament champions with base rates found in samples of professional tennis players; (f) combined different data sets to determine a base rate of left-handedness in the general population; and/or (g) compared top-half ranked players to bottom-half ranked players as a measure of tennis success. For example, Annett (1985) has cited handedness data from Wimbledon: (a) in 1978, 15.6% of the 128 male singles players and 9.4% of the 96 female players were left-handed; and (b) from 1947 through 1978, 15.1% of male champions (5 of 33) and 6.1% of female champions (2 of 33) were left handed. Taken together these findings lend little support for the notion that left-handed professional tennis players have an advantage over their right-handed opponents. The data suggest, however, a possible increased incidence of left-handed racket use in professional male tennis players compared to a large number of young adults which was 8.1% (Annett, 1985, p. 188), and compared to population rates of left-handedness of approximately 10% (Bryden, 1977; Springer and Deutsch, 1989). The findings are quite difficult to interpret, however, because professionals were not allowed to compete at Wimbledon until 1968-the beginning of the four-tournament Open era - and because no other tennis tournaments were examined. Another study (Azemar, Ripoll, Simonet and Stein, 1983) found a higher proportion of left-handed players at specific divisions of the year-end rankings especially those ranked among the top 25 players. However, data were collected from only one year (1980), and females were excluded. Because data from one year may not be representative of actual performance over a longer period of time, and because women were ignored, the robustness of these findings has been appropriately questioned (Wood and Aggleton, 1989).

Others (Wood and Aggleton, 1989) who have examined handedness in professional tennis over a longer time period (viz., 1981, 1986 and 1987) found no overall statistically significant increase in left-handedness compared to population rates of left-handedness for racket use. For male players, however, the rate of left-handedness was consistently higher than the comparative rate of 8.9%, a figure the researchers created by combining data from two studies that used different handedness questionnaires and different populations (viz., Annett, 1970; Bryden, 1977). Left-handed rates of these players ranged from 30% higher (in 1981) to almost 53% higher (in 1987) than the comparison rate. Pooling all male players for all three years, the rate of left-handedness was 37% higher than for the general population (12.2% versus 8.9%). Annett's (1985) more recent rate of left hand racket use (8.1%) been used-rather than combining data from different data sets-the researchers would have found a 43% higher rate of left-handedness in the male players for 1981, a 54% higher rate in 1986, a 68% higher rate in 1987, and a combined rate for all three years to be about 50% higher than the general population. A similar, consistent trend toward increased left-handedness was found in women. The rates of left-handedness for female tennis players ranged from 38.75% higher (in 1981) to 57.5% higher (in 1986) than the comparison rate of 8.0% (the authors noted that data from 1987 were not available for women). Pooling all female players for both years, the rate of left-handedness among tennis professionals was 33.75% higher than for the general population (10.7% versus 8.0%). While combining different data sets to estimate a base rate of left-handedness in the general population is highly questionable, the Wood and Aggleton (1989) study is the only one to date to report rates of left-handedness among tennis professionals for any given year or time frame. Knowing the incidence of left-handedness in as many players as possible at a given point in time is necessary to answer the question of whether there is a left-handed advantage in professional tennis. Once known, the incidence of left-handedness among professional players can be compared with rates found in highly successful players, rather than relying on general population estimates of left-handedness.

Finally, Annett (1985, p. 383) cited data from the 1982 men's tennis tour which suggested a left-handed advantage for male players, based on end-of-the-year computer rankings. Specifically, there were more left-handed male players ranked in the top half than in the bottom half of the rankings. Wood and Aggleton (1989), however, found no such handedness differences when comparing top-half with bottom half ranked male players in 1981, 1986 and 1987. While a top-half versus bottom-half analysis of tennis rankings provides a gross measure of success, bifurcating the rankings is not recommended, because it cannot reveal whether some, but not all, left-handed players evidence a significant superiority in playing professional tennis.

Left-Handedness and Boxing

Boxing is a sport with a long tradition, with roots going back thousands of years to the Olympics of the ancient Greeks (Mullan, 1996). Boxing is a combat sport. In both amateur and professional versions, the fighters wear padded gloves, attacking and defending only with fists. Each round generally lasts for three minutes and the winner is the one who lands the most punches or knocks out his opponent. Boxing is also called pugilism and prizefighting (Mullan, 1996).

There is a common belief that left-handed people are more unskillful. However, the success of the soccer players using their left feet skillfully and the achievements of the artists (Peterson and Lansky, 1974) and tennis (Holtzen, 2000) players are likely the best examples proving the invalidity of this view. It has been reported that there is a high proportion of left-handers among top sportsmen and sportswomen (Azemar et al, 1983; McLean and Cuirczak, 1982). Additionally, it has been suggested that left-handers have an intrinsic advantage over right-handers due to superior spatio-motor skills, and that the relatively high proportion of top left-handed sportsmen and sportswomen is a reflection of this innate superiority. In 1977, a study suggested that approximately 8 to 15% of the adult population was left-handed (Hardyck and Petrinovich, 1977). Tan (1988) reported that the rate of left-handedness was 5% for the Turkish young population. Some studies indicate that left-handedness is more common in males than females (Raymond, Pontier, Dufour, and Pape, 1996; Dane, 2006). Left-handedness, in comparison to the general population, also appears to occur more frequently in identical twins (Cantor et al., 2005), and several groups of neurologically disordered individuals (such as people suffering from epilepsy (Schachter et al., 1995), Down's Syndrome (Batheja and McManus, 1985), autism (Cornish and McManus 1996; Dane and Balci, 2007), mental retardation (Grouios, Sakadami, Poderi, and Alevriadou, 1999), and deafness (Dane and Gumustekin, 2002). Statistically, the identical twin of a left-handed person has a 76% chance of being left-handed, identifying the cause(s) as partly genetic and partly environmental. Also, people of South Asian, Eastern European and Southeast Asian, descent are more likely to be left-handed than any other ethnic group in the world, while people of Western European, Northern European, and African descent are less likely to be left-handed.

The boxing requires a well-disciplined study, strength, a perfect logic, sufficient knowledge, force, and (especially) hand skills of high quality. In the literature we studied on this subject, although there are many studies dealing with the success of boxers, no study has been encountered regarding with the role of hand preference on success in this sport (Johnson, Skorecki, and Wells, 1975; Bianco et al., 2001).

The prevalence of sinistrality in the population has been variously recorded by investigators in many studies at values ranging between 1 and 30%, and approximately 1 in every 10 persons has been reported to be left-handedness (Coren, 1992).

However, in a study made in our region on hand preference in dentistry, this rate was reported to be lower than 30% (Orbak, Tezel, and Tan, 2002). It was determined that 36% of the boxers were left-handed in the National Road Sport Men Boxing Club in Erzurum, Turkey (Gursoy, 2009). These results may be associated with two suggestions: 1. the left-handed subjects have an intrinsic advantage over right-handers due to superior spatio-motor skills, 2. advantage in the left-handed boxer and the left-handed other athletes may result from the nature of the game (boxing) or frequency-dependent strategic advantage.

Annett et al. (1991) stated in their research that hand skill and hand preference were related to the lateralization of cerebral functions, neuromuscular structure and genetic factors. Springer and Deutsch (1998) reported in their study that genetic factors were more effective in determining hand skills, that the probability of the children of right-handed parents was rather low (2%), that in the case that one parent was left-handed this rate was to increase a little (17%), and that if the parents were left-handed the rate would rise more (46%). Although it was stated that hand skill was genetic, showed that hand skill could be improved in time by maintaining some exercises and through motor-learning (Tan, 1993).

A person who is left-handed primarily uses his or her left hand, more so than the right hand; a left-hander will probably use the left hand for tasks such as personal care, cooking, and so on (Kalb, 1976). Writing is not as precise an indicator of handedness as it might seem a better determining of left-handedness results when the differentiation between an individual's major motor activities versus minor or small muscle motor activities is employed. Thus the applications of one's left-hand for eating, writing and similar minor motor activities would be differentiated from major motor activities such as throwing a ball or swinging a bat, etc. While there are numerous individuals who use their left hand for the minor motor activities, there is a much smaller group of people who are "total lefties" i.e. do both minor and major activities with their left hand.

Boxing appears to be something of an exception to the rule that being a southpaw confers an advantage (Mullan, 1996; Sugar, 2007). Until Karl Mildenberger fought Muhammad Ali in 1966, there had not been a southpaw challenger for the heavyweight title since James J Corbett, aka "Gentleman Jim" in 1892, and there have only been three southpaw heavyweight title holders since then: Michael Moorer, Corrie Sanders, and Ruslan Chagaev. However, it is worth distinguishing between the southpaw stances and being left-handed, because some trainers will train a naturally left-handed boxer to fight in an orthodox stance, not merely for convenience but because there may be an advantage in having the jab delivered with the stronger hand. Hence the number of boxers who fought in an orthodox stance may have been converted left-handers. Also in our study that left-handed boxers were more successful than that in the group of right-handedness.

Left-handed people are sometimes placed at a disadvantage by the prevalence of right handed tools in society (Kaya and Orbak, 2004). Many tools and devices are designed to be comfortably used with the right hand. For example, scissors, a very common tool, dental and medical equipments are arranged so that the line being cut along can be seen by a right-handed user, but is obscured to a left-handed user. Furthermore, the handles are often molded in a way that is difficult for a left-hander to hold, and extensive use in such cases can lead to varying levels of discomfort. Dane and Erzurumluoglu (2003) reported that the left-handed handball players had the more advantageous reaction times, or more speed reaction, compared to the right-handed handball players.

Gursoy (2009). The left-handed boxers were found to be more successful than the right-handed ones in the boxing. It was concluded that left-handed athletes may have some neurological advantages and they should never be forced to convert into right-handedness, instead they should be supported both verbally and in terms of equipment and they should be motivated.

References

Annett, J., and Sheridan, M. R. (1973) Effects of S-R and R-R compatibility on bimanual movement time. *Quarterly Journal of Experimental Psychology, 31*, 641-652.

Annett, M. (1970). A classification of hand preference by association analysis. *British Journal of Psychology, 61*, 303–321.

Annett, M. (1985). *Left, right, hand and brain: The right shift theory*. London: Lawrence Erlbaum.

Annett, M. (1991). Laterality and cerebral dominance. *Journal of Child Psychology and Psychiatry, 32*, 219-232.

Azemar, G., Ripoll, H., Simonet, P., and Stein, J. F. (1983). Etude neuropsychologique ducomportement des gauchers en escrime. *Cinesiologie, 22*, 7–18.

Batheja, M., McManus, I. C. (1985). Handedness in the mentally handicapped children. *Developmental Medicine and Child Neurology, 27*, 63–8.

Bisiacchi, P. S., Ripoll, H., Stein, J. F., Simonet, P., and Azemar, G. (1985). Left-handedness in fencers: An attentional advantage? *Perceptual and Motor Skills, 61*, 507–513.

Bradley, J. V. (1957). *Direction of knob–turn stereotypes*. Unites States Air Force, Wright Air Development Center. Technical report.

Brooker, R. J., Lehman, R. A. W. et al. (1981). Hand usage in a colony of bonnet monkeys (Macaca radiata). *Behavior Genetics, 11*, 49-56.

Bryden, M. P. (1977). Measuring handedness with questionnaires. *Neuropsychologia, 15*, 617–624.

Burke, P. H. (1971). Stereophotogrammetric measurement of normal facial asymmetry in children. *Human Biology, 43*, 536-548.

Cantor, J. M, Klassen, P. E., Dickey, R., Christensen, B. K., Kuban, M. E., Blak, T., William, N. S., and Blanchard, R. (2005). Handedness in pedophilia. *Archives of Sexual Behavior. 34*, 447–59.

Chapanis, A., and Gropper, B. A. (1968). The effect of the operator's handedness on some directional stereotypes in control-display relationships. *Human Factors, 10*, 303-320.

Cole, J. (1955). Paw preference in cats related to hand preference in animals and men. *Journal of Comparative and Physiological Psychology, 48*, 137-140.

Collins, R. L. (1969). On the inheritance of handedness: II. Selection for sinistrality in mice. *Journal of Heredity, 60*, 117-119.

Coren S. (1992). *Left-handed everything you need to know about left-handedness.* London: John Murray.

Cornish, K. M., and McManus, I. C. (1996). Hand preference and hand skill in children with autism. *Journal of Autism and Developmental Disorders, 26*, 597–609.

Dane S, and Balci N. (2007). Handedness, eyedness and nasal cycle in children with autism. *International Journal of Developmental Neuroscience, 25*, 223-226.

Dane S. and Erzurumluoglu A. (2003). Sex and handedness differences in eye-hand visual reaction times in handball players. *International Journal of Neuroscience, 113*, 923-929.

Dane, S. (2006). Sex and eyedness in a sample of Turkish high school students. *Perceptual and Motor Skills, 103*, 89-90.

Dane, S., and Bayirli, M. (1998). Correlations between hand preference and durations of hearing for right and left ears in young healthy subjects. *Perceptual and Motor Skills, 86*, 667-672.

Dane, S., and Gumustekin, K. (2002). Handedness in deaf and normal children. *International Journal Neuroscience, 112*, 995-998.

Dane, S., Ersoz, M., Gumustekin, K., Polat, P., and Dastan, A. (2004). Handedness differences in widths of right and left craniofacial regions in healthy young adults. *Perceptual and Motor Skills, 98*, 1261-1264.

Davis, R., Wehrkamp. R., and Smith, K. U. (1951). Dimensional analysis of motion: 1. Effects of laterality and movement direction. *Journal of Applied psychology, 35*, 363-366.

Finch, G. (1941). Chimpanzee handedness. *Science, 94*, 117-118.

Flowers, K. (1975). Handedness and controlled movement. *British Journal of Psychology, 66*, 39-52.

Geschwind, N. and Galaburda, A. (1985a). Cerebral lateralization: Biological mechanisms, associations, and pathology I: A hypothesis and a program for research. *Archives of Neurology, 42*, 428–459.

Geschwind, N. and Galaburda, A. (1985b). Cerebral lateralization: Biological mechanisms, associations, and pathology II: A hypothesis and a program for research. *Archives of Neurology, 42*, 521–552.

Geschwind, N. and Galaburda, A. (1987). *Cerebral lateralization.* Cambridge, MA: MIT Press.

Grant, D. A., and Kaestner, N. F. (1955). Constant velocity tracking as a function of subjects handedness and the rate and drection of the target course. *Journal of Experimental Psychology, 49*, 203-208.

Grondin, S., Guiard, Y., Ivry, R. B. and Coren, S. (1999). Manual laterality and hitting performance in major league baseball. *Journal of Experimental Psychology: Human Perception and Performance, 25*, 747–754.

Grouios, G., Sakadami, N., Poderi, A., and Alevriadou, A. (1999). Excess of non-right handedness among individuals with intellectual disability: Experimental evidence and possible explanations. *Journal of Intellectual Disability* Research, 43, 306–313.

Guatrin, D., and Ettlinger, G. (1970). Lateral preferences in the monkeys. Cortex, 6, 287-292.

Gursoy, R. (2009). *British Journal of Sports Medicine*;43:142-144.

Hardyck, C., and Petrinovich, L. F. (1977). Left-handedness. *Psychological Bulletin, 84*, 385–404.

Holtzen, D. W. (2000). Handedness and professional tennis. *International Journal of Neuroscience, 105*, 101-119.

Johnson, J., Skorecki, J., and Wells, R. P. (1975). Peak accelerations of the head experienced in boxing. *Medical Biological Engineering, 13*, 396-404.

Kalb, B., and Whislgaw. I. (1976). Fundamentals of human neuropsychology (4th ed), W.H. Freemen and Company. New York.

Kaya, M. D., and Orbak, R. (2004). Performance of left-handed dental students is improved when working from the left side of the patient. *International Journal of Industrial Ergonomics, 33*, 387-393.

Keles, P. C., Diyarbakırlı, S., Tan, M., and Tan, U. (1997). Facial asymmetry in right-and left- handed men and women. *International Journal of Neuroscience, 91*, 147-160.

Kimura, D., and Vanderwolf. C. H. (1970). The relation between hand preference and the performance of individual finger movements by left and right hands. *Brain, 93*, 769-774.

McLean, J. M. and Ciurczak, F. M. (1982). Bimanual dexterity in major league baseball players: A statistical study. *New England Journal of Medicine, 307*, 1278–1279.

Milner, A. D. (1969). Distribution of hand preferences in monkeys. *Neuropsychologia, 7*, 375-377.

Mullan, H. (1996). *The ultimate encyclopedia of boxing: The definitive illustrated guide to world boxing*. Edison, NJ: Chartwell Books.

Nass, R. D. and Gazzaniga, M. S. (1987). Cerebral lateralization and specialization in the human central nervous system. In: Plum, F. (Ed.), *Handbook of Physiology: The Nervous System V*. New York: Oxford University Press.

Orbak, R., Tezel, A., and Tan, U. (2002). Right- and left-handed dentists using right- and left-sided dental chairs in treatment of calculus. *International Journal of Neuroscience, 112*, 15-30.

Parlow, S. (1978). Differential finger movements and hand preference. *Cortex, 14*, 608-611.

Peters, M. and Durding, B. (1979). Left-handers and right-handers compared on a motor task. *Journal of Motor Behavior, 11*, 103-111.

Peterson, J., and Lansky, L. (1974). Left handedness among architects. *Perceptual and Motor Skills, 38*, 547-550.

Porac, C., and Coren., S. (1981). *Lateral preference and human behavior*. New York Springer Verlag.

Previc, F. H. (1991). A general theory concerning the prenatal origins of cerebral lateralization in humans. *Psychological Review, 98*, 299-334.

Raymond, M., Pontier, D., Dufour, A., and Pape, M. (1996). Frequency-dependent maintenance of left-handedness in humans, *Proceedings of the Royal Society of London, B. 263*, 1627-1633

Reed, G. F., and Smith, A. C. (1962). A further experimental investigation of the relative speeds of left-and right-handed writers. *Journal of Genetic Psychology, 100*, 275-288.

Simon, J. R. (1964). Steadiness, handedness and hand preference. *Perceptual and Motor Skills, 18*, 203-206.

Simon, J. R., De Crow, T. W., Lincoln, R. S., and Smith, K. U. (1952). Effects of handedness on tracking accuracy. *Perceptual and Motor Skills, 4*, 53-57.

Smith, A. C., and Reed. G. F. (1959). An experimental investigation of the relative speeds of left and right handed writers. *Journal of Genetic Psychology, 94*, 67-76.

Springer, S. P., and Deutsch, G. (1989). *Left brain, right brain (3rd ed.),* New York.

Springer, S. P., and Deutsch, G. (1998). *Left brain, right brain: Perspectives from cognitive neuroscience*. New York: Freeman.

Tan, U. (1988). The distribution of hand preference in normal men and women. *International Journal of Neuroscience, 41*, 35-55.

Tan, U. (1993). Sensory nerve conduction velocities are higher on the left in right hand and motor conduction is faster on the right hand than left in right handed normal subjects. *International Journal of Neuroscience, 73*, 85-91.

Trenouth, M. J. (1985). Asymmetry of the human skull during fetal growth. *The Anatomical Record, 211*, 205-212.

Vig, P. S., and Hewitt, A. B. (1975). Asymmetry of the human facial skeleton. *The Angle Orthodontist, 45*, 125-129.

Warren, J. M. (1953). Handedness in the rhesus monkey. *Science, 118*, 622-623.

Way, E. E. (1958). Relationship of lateral dominance to scores of motor ability and selected skill tests. *Research Quarterly, 29*, 360-369.

Wood, C. J., and Aggleton, J. P. (1989). Handedness in 'fast ball' sports: Do left-handers have an innate advantage? *British Journal of Psychology, 80*, 227 240.

In: Handedness: Theories, Genetics and Psychology ISBN: 978-1-61470-502-4
Editors: J. Dunham and T. Davenport

Chapter VIII

Handedness of Children Determines Preferential Facial and Eye Movements Related to Hemispheric Specialization*

Carmina Arteaga[1,*] ***and Adrián Poblano***[2]
[1]Laboratorio de Neurofisiología Cognoscitiva,
[2]Instituto Nacional de Rehabilitación, Ciudad de México, México

Abstract

Background

Despite repeated demonstrations of asymmetries in several brain functions, the biological bases of such asymmetries have remained obscure The objective of study was to investigate development of lateralized facial

* A version of this chapter also appears in *Brain Mapping and Diseases*, edited by Diane E. Spinelle, published by Nova Science Publishers, Inc. It was submitted for appropriate modifications in an effort to encourage wider dissemination of research.

* Address reprints request: Carmina Arteaga, M.D., M.Sc. Calzada Mexico Xochimilco 289, Col. Arenal Guadalupe, Deleg. Tlalpan, C.P. 14389, Mexico, D.F., Mexico. Pone: (+52) (+55) 59-99-10-00; Fax: (52) (55) 56-03-91-48; E-mail: aeec2001@yahoo.com.mx.

and eye movements evoked by hemispheric stimulation in right-handed and left-handed children.

Methods

Fifty children were tested according to handedness by four tests: I. Mono-syllabic non-sense words, II. Tri-syllabic sense words, III. Visual field occlusion by black wall, and presentation of geometric objects to both hands separatelly, IV. Left eye and the temporal half visual field of the right eye occlusion with special goggles, afterwards asking children to assemble a three-piece puzzle; same tasks were performed contralaterally.

Results

Right-handed children showed higher percentage of eye movements to right side when stimulated by tri-syllabic words, while left-handed children shown higher percentages of eyes movements to left side when stimulated by tri-syllabic words. Left-handed children spent more time in recognizing mono-syllabic words. Hand lateralitycorrelated with tri-syllabic word recognition performance. Age contributed to laterality development in nearly all cases, except in second test.

Conclusions: Eye and facial movements were found to be related to left- and right-hand preference and specialization for language development, as well as visual, haptic perception and recognition in an age-dependent fashion in a very complex process.

Keywords: Handedness, Language, Haptic perception, Visual perception, Left and right hemispheres, Brain specialization

Introduction

Asymmetry in human cerebral hemisphere function, as reflected in a special relationship of the left hemisphere to language, has been recognized for more than a century (Searleman and Porac, 2001). Subsequent observations have identified other aspects of lateralization in brain tasks, such as the superiority of the right hemisphere for spatial manipulations. Despite repeated demonstrations of asymmetries in several functions, the biological bases of such asymmetries have remained obscure (Bear, *et al.,* 1986). This aspect of brain organization, referred to as functional hemispheric asymmetry or functional specialization, is principally noticeable in the human brain (Aboitiz *et al.*, 1995). Most individuals (98 %) show right-hand preference for writing and other manual activities, which are related to cerebral dominance for language in the left hemisphere in 70 % of the cases (Loring *et al.*, 2000). On the other hand, it has been noticed that left-handed subjects have differences in cognitive activities and significant asymmetries when compared with right-handed subjects (Portellano *et al.,* 2006). In the present work, we decided to study lateralization evoked by preferential hemispheric stimuli.

Vision of the human face is an important stimulus for recognizing characteristics of every individual, as well as his/her gender, age and race, and identifying categorical human expressions like: annoyance, happiness, sadness or surprise (Webster *et al.*, 2004). Additionally, it is highly sensitive to identification of several external stimuli, and is related to highly-specialized neural reflexes. Biological motion, especially facial motion, provides a rich and subtle source of information on many tasks, including subject and object recognition, facial speech, and the perception of emotion (Reis and Zaidel, 2001; Hill *et al.,* 2005); however, facial movements have been scarcely studied in relation to specific hemispheric stimulation.

Visual perception depends among other variables, on the form of the object seen. It has been showed that control and visual actions are analyzed in 17 and 18 sensory cortical areas, respectively, when presentation of one object is unidimensional, thus preventing activation of all other areas in the visual cortex (Granel and Goodale, 2003); on the contrary, vision of one object in movement operates 18 and 19 Brodmann areas, respectively. The nasal segment of the visual field of every eye registers the temporal half of the corresponding retina, whereas the temporal region of the visual field registers the nasal half of the retina. In the central nervous system visual pathway, the fibers of the optical nerve that come from the temporal segment of the retina carry information to the same hemisphere, whereas the proceeding ones from the nasal segment of the retina interweave in the optical chiasma and cross to the other hemisphere (Despopoulos and Silbernagl, 1994).

On the other hand, some evidences suggest that eye movements and covert attention may be mediated by complex cognitive mechanisms; for example, cognitive activity produced in one hemisphere can trigger eye movements in the contralateral side (Struthers *et al.* 1992); nonetheless, this evidence requires additional supporting research.

A study performed by Holloway *et al.* (2000) related the sensoriomotor response to hand dominance. Patients were tested by means of sensory-motor hand preference and simultaneous functional Magnetic Resonance Imaging (fMRI), and the authors observed that in the majority of the studied subjects, cortical activation was contralateral to the prefered hand.

Body laterality has distinguished human beings for centuries as a rather exclusive feature of man, in difference with many other species. The causes of this are under research and explanations vary from fetal position during pregnancy to faster maturation of one cerebral hemisphere (Golby *et al.*, 2001). Thus, in this paper, we chose to investigate development in a short life-time period of facial and eye movements evoked by preferential hemispheric stimulation in a sample of right-handed and left-handed healthy school children. Our working hypothesis was: left-handed children have preference for eye and facial movements towards the left side of the face, whereas right-handed children more frequently show eye and facial movements towards the right side, and this effect will depend on age.

Methods

Subjects

The sample was selected from healthy 8 to 10 year-old school-age children. We tested 50 school children from a public school with the following characteristics: age within the range quoted above, each participant demonstrating a normal neurologic examination (Touwen, 1986), with better than 20/20 Snellen visual acuity, normal screening pure-tone audiometry, adequate familial environment (we included only children from integrated families, where both parents lived with the child), middle socio-economic status, and Wechsler Intelligence Scale for Children-Revised in Mexico (WISC-RM Full Scale) over 90 (Wechsler, 1981). Participant did not demonstrate attention deficit-hyperactivity disorder (ADHD), epilepsy, mental retardation, cerebral palsy, or other neurological disorders, psychiatric disorders, congenital malformations (such as those seen in children with Fragile X syndrome) or stuttering. Children were divided in two groups according to handedness (Oldfield, 1971) with the following equation: 100 x ([R-L] / [R+L]) for right- or left-hand use preference. Each group comprised 25 individuals. The Institutional Review Board of the National Institute of Rehabilitation in Mexico City approved the protocol and informed consent and signed forms were obtained from parents and children.

Procedures

We used the experimental design by Zaidel (1984). Children sat comfortably on a chair in front of a desk and were stimulated by means of a word list after Castañeda and Pérez-Ruiz (1991) 20 dB above hearing threshold, and given to the left hemisphere. The list contained the phonetically-balanced most common words used in the Mexico City area. This test is customarily used to obtain word-recognition percentages in Mexico City. Stimuli were delivered biaurally in free-field via loudspeaker using an Amplaid A-171 audiometer (Portland, OR, USA). Children were asked to respond aloud with the correct word, and word types utilized were as follows: Mono-syllabic non-sense, and tri-syllabic sense words (Appendix 1).

Afterwards, the children's vision was occluded by a black wall that covered the full-visual field, and geometric objects were presented separately to each the right or the left hand for haptic hemispheric-prefered recognition. Children were asked to answer in recognition of each object, and correct answers as well as misspellings were recorded (see figure 1).

Next, the left eye and the temporal half visual field of the right eye were occluded with special goggles, and children were requested to assemble a three piece puzzle with the left hand. Afterward, the right eye was occluded as well as the temporal half visual field of the left eye, and the children were asked to perform the same assembly task with the right hand (see figure 2).

All tests were performed begining with the ipsilateral side of the dominant hand in the Edinburg's test. Simultaneous videotape recordings of facial and eye movements while the subject performed each task were employed. Eye and facial movements were visually recorded only by the principal investigator blinded to group pertinance. Videotape recordings were conducted with the video camera located in front of the face at level of the nose, with the face uncovered and clean, without hair or glasses and with adequate brightness. Facial and eye movements in each test were evaluated using frame-by-frame slow motion of film recordings of 333-msec periods (Video Camera Recorder CCD-TR350, Sony Corporation, Tokio, Japan), in a VHS-HQ DA4 videocassette player (Goldstar, Seoul, Korea) in a JVC TV monitor (JVC, New Jersey, USA). Variables studied included the following: stretching of the mouth, (depressor *labii inferioris* movements, and elevation of *labii superioris, orbicularis oris,* and the zygomatic muscles) and lateral eye movements (*rectus internus oculi,rectus externus oculi, obliquus* superior muscle and *obliquus* inferior muscle) as binomial variables. No movements of the frontal region were observed during performance of four tests; therefore, none were included in the analysis. Subsequently, the latencies of each movement were calculated employing frame-by-frame analysis as continuous variables.

Statistical Analysis

The mean and standard deviation (SD) of quantitative variables and the percentages of binomial variables were calculated. Kruskal-Wallis test was used to compare binomial variables frequency (percentages of eye movements to right and left side; and percentages of labial right and left movements). In addition, we compared quantitative variable averages were compared using Student's *t* test (eye and facialmovements latencies in each condition). Logistic regression was used to investigate the influence of hand laterality on each test performance. ANOVA for repeated measurements was used, utilizing the test type as a level-four factor for each year of age of children and employing Huynh-Feldt corrections for homosedasticity assessment. The *p* value accepted *a priori* for detecting differences was $p \leq 0.05$.

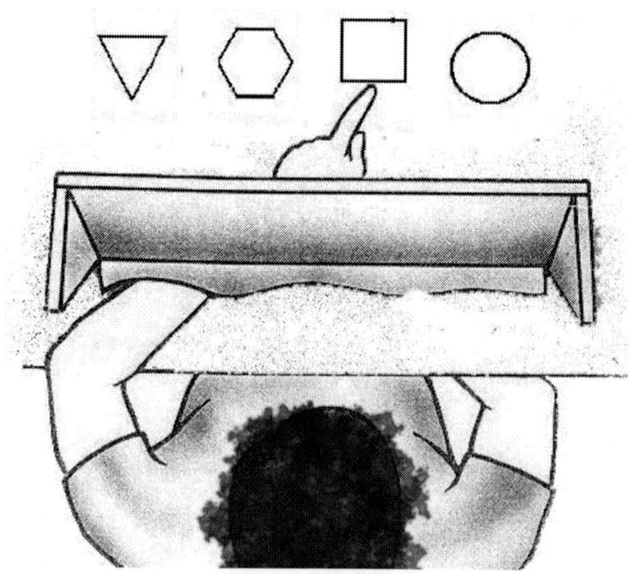

Figure 1. Design of the Haptic Recognition Test. Subject's visual field was occluded by the black wall. The subject was asked to recognized figures with each hand.

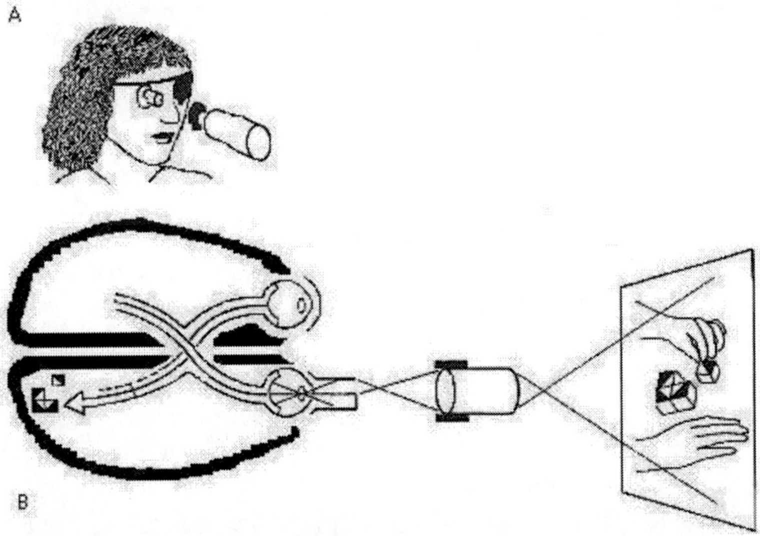

Figure 2. Selective Hemi-field Visual Recognition Test. Contralateral eye and temporal visual field was occluded while the subject used only the nasal hemi-field for puzzle assembly. A. Design of special goggles. B. Visual pathway between stimuli and occipital visual cortex.

Results

Twelve male and 13 female right-handed children were analyzed, while the left-handed group consisted of 11 male and 14 female children. Mean (± standard deviation, SD) of age of right-handed children was 100.96 ± 10.83 months and of left-handed children, 109.76 ± 11.50 months. Average of Edinburgh test quotients of right-handed children was 84.4, while of left-handed children was 22.

Percentages in each sub-test of preferent hemispheric stimulation yielded significant differences between both groups of children in discrimination of the tri-syllabic word test when comparing right and left eye movements, right-handed children demonstrated higher discrimination percentages (see Table I). Latencies of facial and eye movements in each preferent hemispheric stimulation sub-test are shown in Table II. Left-handed children spent significantly more time in recognizing mono-syllabic words ($t = -2.03$, $p = 0.048$).

Using logistic regression, hand laterality correlated only with recognition of tri-syllabic words (r = .489, $p = 0.027$). In ANOVA tests, we found evidenced for significant contribution of age to laterality within subjects in the mono-syllabic recognition test (F = 4.52, df = 1, 4.62, $p = 0.041$), geometrical figure recognition in the contralateral hand test ($F = 6.16$, $df = 1, 6.22$, $p = 0.018$), and puzzle assembly in the contralateral vision field test ($F = 5.30$, $df = 1, 5.60$, $p = 0.027$).

Discussion

As can be seen in Table I, right-handed children exhibited higher percentages of eye movements to the right side when stimulated by tri-syllabic words, while left-handed children demonstrated higher percentages of eye movements to the left side when stimulated by tri-syllabic words. Left-handed children spent more time in recognizing mono-syllabic non-sense words (Table II). Hand laterality correlated with tri-syllabic word recognition performance. Age contributed significantly to laterality development in nearly all tests with the exception of the tri-syllabic word recognition test.

Right-handed children showed higher percentages of eye movements to the right side, with specialization of left hemisphere in language decoding. Many research articles support left hemisphere dominance for language recognition, including Steinmetz *et al.,* (1991), who showed that *planum temporale* asymmetry correlated with hand dominance. On the other hand, left-handed individuals had a lesser degree of leftward asymmetry than right-handed individuals, as measured by magnetic resonance imaging (MRI). Recently Mäkelä *et al.* (2005) studied N-100 magnetoencephalographic (MEG) responses to constant-formant vowels and diphthongs with formant transitions: all the stimuli elicited prominent auditory N-100 responses, but the formant transitions resulted in latency modulations specific to the left hemisphere. As expected from a review of the literature and the investigations quoted above, left dominance for language in right-handed children induced more right-side eye movements when sense words were used as stimuli; contrariwise, left-handed children showed greater frequency of left-side eye movements for language stimuli as a result of their incomplete left-hemisphere dominance for speech processing (Struthers *et al.* 1992).

The longer time used in mono-syllabic non-sense words recognition by left-handed children may be attributed to incomplete left-hemisphere specialization and difficulties for mastering language, verbal fluency, or linguistic-processing speed, as has been proposed for children with language delay and developmental learning disorders (Poblano *et al.* 2000; Herbert *et al.* 2005). Although the left-handed children studied are asymptomatic and exhibit good school performance, which suggest that this group of children is at high risk for language-reading difficulties. On the other hand, Knetch *et al.* (2001) suggested that atypical hemispheric specialization for language is not associated with major impairments of linguistic faculties in healthy subjects; thus, additional research is need to lend support to this finding.

Hand laterality correlated with word recognition. This fact confirms previous data from the literature supporting the role of left-hemisphere specialization for language dominance, as shown by Wyllie *et al.* (1990) utilizing intracarotid amobarbital administration in the language-dominance test and its correlation with cortical stimulation, and by Schwartz, *et al,* (1996) during recordings of electroencephalographic activity after craniotomy of right-handed patients with epilepsy.

Hand-preference development has been shown to be age-dependent, especially in the earlier stages of childhood. For example, Curt *et al.* (1992), found in 765 pre-school children that hand-asymmetry distribution for one moving task and for a graphic test was mainly age-dependent.

Development of handedness and lateralization, and the relationships of these abilities to additional bodily functions, is a complex and not well-known process. For example, auditory perception and its relationship to other lateralized functions is not well known, but deserves more attention in future research.

This study presents some limitations, including the low number of subjects studied, and the cross-sectional study design employed, which could have been improved by the use of a prospective follow-up. These points merit additional attention in future works. Notwithstanding this, we learned that interactions between lateralization of eye and facial movements is a complex, age-influenced process, a process wich will be studied in greater detail in future works.

Acknowledgment

The authors' thanks go to Lucia Vega B.Sc., Principal of the Republic of Swaziland School, for her help in this research and to Maggie Brunner, M.A., and Eduardo Castro-Sierra Ph.D. for their comments and help in the preparation of the English version of the paper.

References

Aboitiz, F., Ide, A., Navarrete, A., Peña, M., Rodríguez, E., Wolf, V., and Zaidel, E. (1995) The anatomical substrate for language and hemispheric specialization. *Biological Reviews.* 28: 45-50.

Bear, D., Schiff, D., Saver, J., Greenberg, M., and Freeman, R. (1986) Quantitative analysis of cerebral asymmetries. Fronto-occipital correlation, sexual dimorphism, and association with handedness. *Archives of Neurology.* 43: 598-603.

Castañeda, G.R., and Pérez-Ruiz, S.J. (1991) Phonetic analysis of common use-word lists in speech audiometry (in Spanish). *Otorrinolaringologia Mexicana.*36: 23-30.

Curt, F., Maccario, J., and Dellatolas, G. (1992) Distribution of hand preference and hand skill asymmetry in preschool children: theoretical implications. *Neuropsychologia*. 30: 27-34.

Despopoulos, A., and Silbernagl, S. (1994) *Text and atlas of physiology.* (in Spanish). Barcelona. Mosby/Doyma. pp. 300 – 310.

Golby, J.A., Poldrack, R.A., Brewer, J.B., Spencer, D., Desmond, J.E., Aron, A.P., and Gabrieli, J.D.E. (2001) Material-specific lateralization in the medial temporal lobe and prefrontal cortex during memory ecoding . *Brain.* 123: 1841-1854.

Granel, T., Goodale, M.A. (2003) Visual control of action but not perception requires analytical processing of object shape. *Nature.* 426: 664 - 667.

Herbert, M.R., Ziegler, D.A., Deutsch, C.K., O'Brien, L.M., Kennedy, D.N., Filipek, P.A., Bakardjiev, A.I., Hodgson, J., Takeoka, M., Makris, N., and Caviness, V.S.Jr. (2005) Brain asymmetries in autism and developmental language disorder: a nest whole-brain analysis. *Brain.* 128: 213-226.

Hill, H.C.H., Troje, N.F., and Johnston, A. (2005) Range- and domain- specific exaggeration of facial speech. *Journal of Vision.* 5: 793-807.

Holloway, V., Gadian, D.G., Vargha-Khadem, F., Porter, D.A., Boyd, S.G., and Connelly, A. (2000) The reorganization of sensorimotor function in children after hemispherectomy. *Brain.* 123:2432-2444.

Knecht, S., Dräger, B., Flöel, A., Lohman, H., Breittenstein, C., Deppe, M., Henningsen, H., and Ringelstein E.-B. (2001) Behavioral relevance of atypical language lateralization in healthy subjects. *Brain.* 124: 1657-1665.

Loring, D.W., Meador, K.J., Allison, J.D., and Wright, J.C. (2000) Relationship between motor and language activation using fMRI. *Neurology.* 54: 981-983.

Mäkelä, A.M., Alku, P., May, P. J. C., Mäkinen, V., and Tiitinen, H. (2005) left-hemispheric brain activity reflects format transitions in speech sounds. *Neuroreport.* 16: 549-553.

Oldfield, R.C. (1971) The assessment and analysis of handedness: The Edinburgh inventory. *Neuropsychologia.* 9: 97-113.

Poblano, A., Valadez-Tepec, T., Arias, M.L., García-Pedroza, F. (2000) Phonological and visuo-spatial working memory alterations in dyslexic children. *Arch. Med. Res.*31: 493-496.

Portellano, J.A., Torrijos, S., Martínez-Arias, R., and Vale, P. (2006) Cognitive performance of right handed and left-handed persons on the Wechsler adult intelligence scale (WAIS-III). *Rev. Neurol.* 42: 73-76.

Reis, V.A., and Zaidel, D.W. (2001) Brain and face: communicating signals of health in the left and right sides of the face. *Brain and Cognition.* 46: 240-244.

Schwartz, T.H., Ojeman, G.A., Haglund, M.M., and Lettich, E. (1996) Cerebral lateralization of neuronal activity during naming, reading and line-matching. *Cognitive Brain Research.* 4: 263-273.

Searleman, A., and Porac, C. (2001) Lateral preference patterns as posible correlates of successfully switched left hand writing: data and a theory. *Laterality.* 6: 303-314.

Steinmetz, H., Volkman, J., Jänke, L., and Freund, H-J. (1991) Anatomical left-right asymmetry of language-related temporal cortex is different in left- and right-handers. *Annals of Neurology.* 29: 315-319.

Struthers, G., Charlton, S., and Bakan, P. (1992) Lateral orientation, eye movements and dichotic listening. *International Journal of Neurosciences.* 66: 189-195.

Touwen, B.C.L. (1986). *The neurological examination of the child with minor nervous dysfunction.* (in Spanish). Buenos Aires Panamericana.

Webster, M.A., Kaping, D., Mizokami, Y., and Duhamel, P. (2004) Adaptation to natural facial categories. *Nature.* 428: 557-561.

Weschler, D. (1981) *WISC-R Scale of intelligence revised for school level.*(in Spanish) Mexico City, Manual Moderno.

Wyllie, E., Lüders, H., Murphy, D., Morris, H., Dinner, D., Lesser, R., Godoy, J., Kotagal, P., and Kanner, A. (1990) Intracarotid amobarbital (Wada) test for language dominance: correlation with results of cortical stimulation. *Epilepsia.* 3: 156-161.

Zaidel, D.W. (1984) The functions of the right hemisphere (in Spanish). *La Recherche.* 4: 504-513.

Index

C

D

E

F

G

H

I

N

O

P

Q

R

S

T

U

V